Multiple Choice Questions for Primary Health Care

This book is dedicated to Professor Brian McGuinness, with grateful thanks for his personal energy and enthusiasm for excellence in clinical education and primary care.

Multiple Choice Questions for Primary Health Care
second edition

Amanda Howe, Christopher Hand, Mei Ling Denney and Judith Neaves

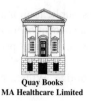

Quay Books
MA Healthcare Limited

Quay Books Division, MA Healthcare Limited, Jesses Farm, Snow Hill, Dinton,
Salisbury, Wiltshire, SP3 5HN

British Library Cataloguing-in-Publication Data
A catalogue record is available for this book

© MA Healthcare Limited 2005
ISBN 1 85642 244 5

Printed by Cromwell Press, Trowbridge, Wiltshire

Contents

Foreword

The endpoint of medical education is a safe and effective medical practitioner. Such an individual can be identified only by a process of assessment. There has been a welcome change in the approach to assessment in medical education over the past thirty years with more emphasis on the candidate's ability to carry out the tasks associated with being a doctor and less emphasis on the recall of the minutiae of knowledge (so which enzyme does catalyse the fourth reaction in Kreb's Cycle?). Nevertheless, there is a continuing need for a sound knowledge base to underpin performance. Indeed, there is a direct correlation between measures of knowledge and clinical performance.

The multiple choice question (MCQ) is a useful tool for rapidly assessing factual recall. Because the scoring is clear cut, it is particularly suited for use as a self-assessment tool. Unfortunately, the format lends itself to the examination of trivia, with one early instruction manual on writing MCQs suggesting opening a standard textbook at random and picking the first topic encountered.

The current collection has avoided this pitfall. It is based around a systematically planned core curriculum that should meet the needs of undergraduates and postgraduates wishing to take a general overview of their own knowledge. The questions concentrate on factual clinical knowledge rather the complexities of decision-making, application and areas of judgement. This is not because the authors think that these areas are unimportant, but because the MCQ is not the best way of assessing them. This book will allow you to assess whether you have the range of basic knowledge needed to support the complex decisions you will need to take in formal examinations and in your future clinical practice.

Professor Sam Leinster
Dean of the School of Medicine, Health Policy and Practice,
University of East Anglia
2004

Preface

The opportunity to prepare a second edition of 'MCQs in Primary Care' was given to me by the author of the first edition, Professor Brian McGuinness, an erudite and hard working colleague whose reputation as one of the founding influences on UK academic general practice is well established. He approached me because of my association with one of the newest medical schools in England, in the hope that the material in this text would be of value for those training the doctors of tomorrow. I invited other colleagues to co-author the second edition, mainly because most works are strengthened by input from more than one person's expertise, but also because, even in the short period since the book's original publication, the state of clinical knowledge has moved on, and all the evidence base for the questions had to be reviewed.

We have taken considerable steps to modernise the text, matching the questions to the common problems which underpin clinical practice, and which therefore constitute the knowledge needed by anyone practising in a primary care setting. The book is aimed particularly at medical undergraduates, postgraduate trainees for primary care, those still in training whose career path is as yet unclear, and any health worker wanting to review their factual knowledge.

The authors have had to make choices — identifying reliable sources that would be accessible to most readers; confining ourselves to the kind of material that is likely to remain 'current' (thus avoiding questions on specific UK policies such as the 'National Service Frameworks'); and accepting that some readers will disagree with our interpretations of source material. We have done our best to ensure that the information is accurate. We hope it will be useful.

It is no mistake that all the authors are practising GPs and educationalists, as they can bring both a general overview of clinical practice and a detailed appreciation of the levels of knowledge needed by the target audience. I would personally like to thank my co-authors Mei Ling Denney, Christopher Hand, and Judith Neaves for all their hard work and collegial support; Professor Brian McGuinness for generously offering us the opportunity to take over the authorship; the Royal College of General Practitioners East Anglia Faculty for helping with the identification of suitable co-authors; the GP representatives on the UEA 'Unit Teams' for their help in peer review of the questions; and the Dean of the School of Medicine, Health Policy and Practice, Sam Leinster, for his advice and help.

Professor Amanda Howe
Professor of Primary Care
School of Medicine, Health Policy and Practice,
University of East Anglia
2004

List of conventional terms

Throughout the book, a number of descriptive terms have been used. In order that the reader may understand the meanings of certain conventional terms which appear frequently, these are listed below:

Pathognomonic, Diagnostic, Characteristic, Cardinal imply that a feature would occur in at least 90% of cases.

Typically, Frequently, Significantly, Commonly, In general often imply that a feature would occur in at least 60% of cases.

In the majority implies that a feature occurs in greater than 50% of cases.

In the minority implies that a feature occurs in less than 50% of cases.

Low chance, Marginal and *In a substantial minority* imply that a feature may occur in less than 30% of cases.

Has been shown, Recognised, Reported and *Associated with* all refer to evidence which can be found in an authoritative medical text. None of these terms makes any implication about the frequency with which the feature occurs.

Some terms have been taken from the advice available to candidates taking the MRCGP examination, for which grateful acknowledgement is made.

Part 1
Multiple choice questions

Introduction

Historically, most medical examinations have included multiple choice questions (MCQs) as their main test of clinical knowledge. From the assessment point of view, the main advantage of multiple choice 'true/false' questions is their conciseness. Students can answer the questions quickly, so the test can cover a broad domain. They are very valuable as a self-assessment tool, and are often used formatively to check progress towards acquiring a certain level of factual knowledge.

The material for the MCQ sections has been based on the planned core clinical curriculum of a modern medical course, and is organised by systems. Even a text with more than 200 questions will only begin to touch on the full breadth of knowledge which is useful to clinicians. We have taken the perspective of the generalist, and confined questions mostly to common conditions about which anyone practising in primary care would need to have some grasp, and about which junior doctors would need to have some knowledge.

MCQs do have their limitations. Clinicians will always debate the generalisability of facts, and will usually be sceptical of precise facts and figures since their experiences will often show them the exception to any rule. Knowledge in medicine changes fast, even in matters of 'fact', such as the prevalence of a disease, or the best use of a common technical investigation. In addition, many facts can be quickly retrieved from information sources, and the need to 'store' such information in one's brain is less if rapid access via electronic means is available. Nevertheless, the practice of clinical medicine is complex, and the need to act efficiently and effectively requires practitioners to be able to recall and use a large amount of knowledge without recourse to reference material. MCQs are therefore a way of testing that such knowledge is 'at your fingertips' ie. that you can retrieve it quickly and accurately when needed.

Some aspects of clinical practice do not lend themselves to MCQs. Describing the principles of effective interprofessional teamworking, or testing appropriate communication skills, generally require other modalities, as MCQ format would render such complex interpersonal processes banal. For example, try 'effective consultation with a patient requires the doctor to hold eye contact for a minimum of 30% of the time' — questions immediately arise as to what type of consultation, what 'eye contact' means, whether this is true in all cultures and so on.... perhaps a shy patient would find 30% excessive, whereas a confident assertive person would find it too little. For this reason, many social science aspects of clinical knowledge are not included in the examples given in this book, as the margins of interpretation are too great.

Assessors may vary in how they score MCQs, and it is important that candidates know how the papers will be marked, as this will vary their approach. If wrong answers are negatively marked, then guessing is more hazardous than leaving some questions unanswered. In order to encourage readers to self-test rigorously, we have put the answers at the end of the book, rather than beneath each answer.

Section 1

Being a doctor, being a patient

1.1 In febrile seizures   T   F

(a) Around 4% of children are affected   □ □

(b) The probability of bacterial meningitis is high   □ □

(c) After the first febrile seizure, recurrence is highest in the one to three age group   □ □

(d) Prophylactic treatment decreases the likelihood of future seizures   □ □

(e) Duration of seizure is usually less than fifteen minutes and frequency not more than once in twenty-four hours   □ □

1.2 Measles, mumps and rubella vaccination (MMR)

(a) There is good evidence linking MMR with autism   □ □

(b) It is given at thirteen months and at pre-school entry   □ □

(c) 10% of children develop fever, malaise, and rash five to twenty-one days after the first immunisation   □ □

(d) More than 95% of children need to be immunised to obtain herd immunity   □ □

(e) Mild egg allergy is a contraindication   □ □

1.3 The following are diseases

    □ □

(a) Ageing

    □ □

(b) Childbirth and pregnancy

    □ □

(c) Unhappiness

    □ □

	T	F

(d) Baldness ☐ ☐

(e) Jetlag ☐ ☐

1.4 Nurse practitioners in primary care

(a) Have longer consultations than doctors ☐ ☐

(b) Order fewer investigations than doctors ☐ ☐

(c) Have consultations that result in greater patient satisfaction compared to those with doctors ☐ ☐

(d) Can prescribe many of the same drugs as doctors ☐ ☐

(e) Can provide equivalent care to doctors ☐ ☐

1.5 Investigations in clinical practice

(a) Are, in general, overused ☐ ☐

(b) Are starting to decline in terms of numbers ☐ ☐

(c) 5% of test results are outside the reference range ☐ ☐

(d) Are performed more appropriately if guidelines are issued ☐ ☐

(e) Have higher levels of sensitivity and specificity in primary care than in secondary care ☐ ☐

1.6 Care of the dying

(a) Very few patients now die with uncontrolled symptoms ☐ ☐

(b) More people die at home than in hospices ☐ ☐

(c) Heart failure is a very common cause of death in hospital medical wards ☐ ☐

(d) Inability to take drugs by mouth makes symptom control extremely difficult ☐ ☐

T   F

(e) Taking morphine as required is better than taking it regularly due to the risk of addiction ☐ ☐

1.7 Tetanus

(a) Remains a public health problem throughout the developing world ☐ ☐

(b) Toxin blocks the inhibition of GABA to motor neurones ☐ ☐

(c) Only occurs in obviously contaminated wounds ☐ ☐

(d) Primary prevention can be achieved using a live vaccine ☐ ☐

(e) Can occur in the neonate ☐ ☐

1.8 Physical activity

(a) Has been shown to improve quality of life ☐ ☐

(b) Has no effect on the symptoms of depression ☐ ☐

(c) Is associated with osteoporosis ☐ ☐

(d) Is of little benefit in peripheral arterial disease ☐ ☐

(e) Can be increased effectively by counselling patients in primary care ☐ ☐

1.9 Bacterial meningitis

(a) In children has fallen in incidence by 30%, following the introduction of conjugate Haemophilus influenzae B (Hib) vaccines ☐ ☐

(b) In infants confers a significantly greater risk of learning disability and neuromotor function ☐ ☐

(c) If suspected in a child, should be treated with benzylpenicillin syrup before the child is sent to hospital ☐ ☐

(d) When caused by pneumococcal and haemophilus infections should be treatment with cefotaxime as the drug of first choice ☐ ☐

(e) Is most commonly caused by Neisseria meningitides ☐ ☐

1.10 The following are recognised as work-related diseases

T   F

(a) Leptospirosis

(b) Mesothelioma

(c) Presbycusis

(d) Vibration white finger

(e) Tietze's disease

1.11 The following factors have been shown to be closely related to compliance with advice and treatment in general practice

(a) Severity of symptoms

(b) Age and sex

(c) Continuity of doctor

(d) Higher qualifications of doctor

(e) Short waiting time for appointment

1.12 The following deaths should be reported to the coroner

(a) When the death occurred during an operation or before recovery from an anaesthetic

(b) When the patient has had no medical care for at least three months

(c) When the patient was suffering from a registered industrial disability

(d) When the patient has a pacemaker *in situ*

(e) When the patient has had radiotherapy within the last six months

1.13 Recognised complications of infectious mononucleosis include

(a) Facial palsy

(b) Thrombocytopaenia

	T	F
(c) Pericarditis	☐	☐
(d) Glomerulonephritis	☐	☐
(e) Agammaglobulinaemia	☐	☐

1.14 The following infectious diseases are notifiable

	T	F
(a) Rubella	☐	☐
(b) Exanthema subitum	☐	☐
(c) Typhoid	☐	☐
(d) Measles	☐	☐
(e) Meningitis	☐	☐

1.15 The following have a well-established relationship with chronic cigarette smoking

	T	F
(a) Increased incidence of bladder cancer	☐	☐
(b) Increased perinatal mortality rate	☐	☐
(c) Peptic ulcer incidence	☐	☐
(d) Decreased serum IgE	☐	☐
(e) Raised blood pressure	☐	☐

1.16 The following conditions are recognised X-linked recessive disorders

	T	F
(a) Duchenne muscular dystrophy	☐	☐
(b) Haemophilia	☐	☐
(c) Glucose 6 PD deficiency	☐	☐
(d) Marfan's syndrome	☐	☐
(e) Down's syndrome	☐	☐

1.17 In the routine application of epidemiology to clinical practice T F

(a) Point prevalence tends to underestimate the total frequency of a chronic condition ☐ ☐

(b) The incidence rate is the proportion of a defined group developing a condition within a stated period ☐ ☐

(c) Within-observer variation is largely random ☐ ☐

(d) Random subject variation is not associated with regression to the mean ☐ ☐

(e) The validity of a screening test is measured by comparing its performance with a reference test ☐ ☐

1.18 Haemophilus influenzae type B immunisation

(a) Is a live viral vaccine ☐ ☐

(b) Preterm babies should be immunised according to chronological age ☐ ☐

(c) Protects against non-invasive Hib diseases such as otitis media ☐ ☐

(d) Should not be given at the same time as DTP vaccine ☐ ☐

(e) No booster doses are required after a primary course ☐ ☐

1.19 Legal requirements of a doctor completing Form C in an application for cremation are to

(a) Be registered for at least five years from date of provisional registration ☐ ☐

(b) Be unrelated to the deceased ☐ ☐

(c) Have examined the body after death and questioned the doctor completing Form B ☐ ☐

(d) Be unrelated to and not in partnership with the doctor completing Form B ☐ ☐

(e) Have informed the coroner within forty-eightl hours of the death ☐ ☐

1.20 Patients with no spleen or severe dysfunction of the spleen should be immunised against

		T	F
(a)	Haemophilus influenzae type B (Hib)	☐	☐
(b)	Meningococcus types B and C	☐	☐
(c)	Influenza	☐	☐
(d)	Tetanus	☐	☐
(e)	Pneumococcal disease	☐	☐

Section 2

Locomotion

2.1 In a middle-aged patient with acute back pain   T   F

  (a) The most likely cause is subluxation of the apophyseal joints   ☐ ☐

  (b) Wasting of the thigh muscles indicates an L5 nerve root lesion   ☐ ☐

  (c) Laminectomy will relieve back pain due to instability   ☐ ☐

  (d) Bilateral sciatica may be an indication of a cauda equina lesion   ☐ ☐

  (e) Degenerative spondylolisthesis is usually of L4 or L5   ☐ ☐

2.2 Restless legs syndrome

  (a) Is more prevalent in patients with fibromyalgia and those with rheumatoid arthritis   ☐ ☐

  (b) Is associated with diagnostic abnormalities found on clinical examination   ☐ ☐

  (c) May be treated with clonazepam, carbamazepine, or levodopa   ☐ ☐

  (d) Affects men and women equally at any age   ☐ ☐

  (e) Has symptoms which are alleviated by activity   ☐ ☐

2.3 When considering minor orthopaedic problems of childhood

  (a) 90% of all cases of metatarsus varus spontaneously resolve by the age of four   ☐ ☐

  (b) Flat feet that are normal can be distinguished from those that are abnormal by asking the child to stand on tiptoe   ☐ ☐

  (c) In a pre-school child with knock knees, 15cm of intermalleolar separation is acceptable   ☐ ☐

T   F

(d) Tibia vara is more common in West Indian children   ☐ ☐

(e) 'Squinting patellae' are a typical finding in persistent femoral anteversion   ☐ ☐

2.4 Developmental dysplasia of the hip (DDH) is more likely in children

(a) With family history of DDH   ☐ ☐

(b) Following a breech delivery   ☐ ☐

(c) Of northern European parentage   ☐ ☐

(d) With foot deformities   ☐ ☐

(e) With reduced range of adduction   ☐ ☐

2.5 Considering childhood disorders of bone and joint, the following statements apply

(a) Osteogenesis imperfecta may present late, during adolescence   ☐ ☐

(b) Osteomyelitis is a recognised feature of Osgood Schlatter syndrome   ☐ ☐

(c) Osteoid osteoma is usually a painless condition   ☐ ☐

(d) Males are at greater risk of talipes equinovarus   ☐ ☐

(e) Prognosis in Marfan's disease is determined by degree of spinal deformity   ☐ ☐

2.6 In soft tissue, corticosteroid injections

(a) There is good evidence from RCTs to support their use   ☐ ☐

(b) Can improve trigger finger   ☐ ☐

(c) If done directly into a tendon can cause rupture of the tendon   ☐ ☐

(d) Are contraindicated in patients under twenty   ☐ ☐

(e) Sepsis is not a recognised complication   ☐ ☐

2.7 Hip fracture

		T	F
(a)	Antibiotic prophylaxis before surgery is beneficial	☐	☐
(b)	Postoperative prophylaxis with heparin or antiplatelet agents is usual	☐	☐
(c)	Is more common in men than women	☐	☐
(d)	Is usually sustained through a fall from standing height or less	☐	☐
(e)	One in five people die in the first year afterwards	☐	☐

2.8 Radiography in primary care patients with low back pain of at least six weeks' duration is associated with

(a)	Greater patient satisfaction	☐	☐
(b)	Improved patient functioning	☐	☐
(c)	Reduced doctor workload	☐	☐
(d)	Improved severity of pain	☐	☐
(e)	A high yield of findings that alter clinical management	☐	☐

2.9 Back pain

(a)	When acute is best treated with minimal rest and rapid return to normal activity	☐	☐
(b)	Psychological and behavioural responses to pain and social factors are the main determinants of chronic pain and disability	☐	☐
(c)	Psychological treatments in pain management programmes are ineffective	☐	☐
(d)	Addressing patients' beliefs and coping strategies are an integral part of management	☐	☐
(e)	The majority become increasingly incapacitated	☐	☐

2.10 Symptoms of paraesthesiae

T   F

(a) Are diagnostic of carpal tunnel syndrome if reproduced by Phalen's test

(b) With ulnar nerve palsy may indicate need for nerve transplantation

(c) Are a common feature of Raynaud's Syndrome

(d) Are typically linked with endocrine disorders

(e) Can be caused by vitamin deficiency

2.11 Ankle and foot injuries

(a) Acute ankle sprains are associated with fractures in more than 25% of cases

(b) With inability to weight bear is an indication for radiography

(c) Tenderness of the base of the fifth metatarsal is an indication for X-ray

(d) A fracture of the mid-foot is commonly associated with tenderness of the calcaneum

(e) Tenderness of the posterior edge of the medial malleolus is associated with fracture of the fibula

2.12 *Cauda equina* syndrome

(a) Is frequently due to lumbar disc prolapse

(b) May present with impotence

(c) Constitutes a medical emergency

(d) Can be of gradual onset over a period of weeks

(e) Typically includes urinary retention

2.13 Manual therapy

		T	F

(a) Is more effective for acute neck pain than conventional physiotherapy ☐ ☐

(b) Has been shown to be beneficial in chronic low back pain ☐ ☐

(c) Is contraindicated in inflammatory arthritides ☐ ☐

(d) Is less effective than non steroidal anti–inflammatory drugs in acute back pain ☐ ☐

(e) Is less costly than physiotherapy for acute neck pain ☐ ☐

2.14 In work-related disorders

(a) In repetitive strain injury there is usually a history of injury at the start of the illness ☐ ☐

(b) Acute injuries at work account for less than 50% of work related illness ☐ ☐

(c) Carpal tunnel syndrome can be a repetitive strain injury ☐ ☐

(d) The risk of repetitive strain injury at a computer is reduced by working in one position that is ergonomically designed ☐ ☐

(e) The employer is responsible for supplying wrist splints and other aids if required ☐ ☐

2.15 Carpal tunnel syndrome

(a) Is an uncommon cause of hand pain at night ☐ ☐

(b) Can affect the ring finger ☐ ☐

(c) Incidence peaks in men at age forty-five to fifty-five ☐ ☐

(d) It is recognised that cycling provokes symptoms ☐ ☐

(e) 34% will resolve with no treatment over six months ☐ ☐

2.16 In osteoarthritis   T   F

(a) There is a strong geographical association   ☐   ☐

(b) There is an uncertain association with osteoporosis   ☐   ☐

(c) Osteoarthritis of the hip is more common in females   ☐   ☐

(d) Knee osteoarthritis is associated with farming   ☐   ☐

(e) Heberden's nodes start as cysts filled with hyaluronate ☐   ☐

2.17 In osteoarthritis

(a) Subchondral cysts are areas of reduced mechanical stress ☐   ☐

(b) Chondroitin levels increase in cartilage   ☐   ☐

(c) The chondrocyte has oestrogen receptors   ☐   ☐

(d) Paracetamol is an effective management option   ☐   ☐

(e) Chondroitin is not an effective treatment   ☐   ☐

Section 3

Blood and skin

3.1 Athlete's foot   T   F

  (a) Does not involve toe nails   □ □

  (b) Is more common in swimming pool users and industrial workers   □ □

  (c) Is present in 15% of the population   □ □

  (d) Can spread to other parts of the body   □ □

  (e) Is best treated with oral rather than topical preparations   □ □

3.2 Pressure ulcers

  (a) Are the third costliest disorder after cancer and cardiovascular disorders   □ □

  (b) Occur in up to 30% of patients admitted to hospital   □ □

  (c) Can be prevented by measures that are inexpensive and not labour intensive   □ □

  (d) Risk assessment scales are of limited effectiveness   □ □

  (e) Can be prevented by pressure reducing mattresses   □ □

3.3 Blood transfusion

  (a) Human error causes morbidity and mortality that is preventable   □ □

  (b) There is now no risk of transmission of HIV, or hepatitis B and C   □ □

  (c) Half of all blood transfused in the UK is to surgical patients   □ □

  (d) The need can be reduced by careful planning of patient care   □ □

T   F

(e) Blood substitutes are likely to replace blood transfusions in the near future ☐ ☐

3.4 Children below the age of one with atopic eczema
☐ ☐

(a) Commonly show areas of purpura that are due to scratching

(b) Typically have facial involvement ☐ ☐

(c) Are more likely to be allergic to house dust mite than to food substances ☐ ☐

(d) Should routinely be prescribed a suitable emollient for twice daily use ☐ ☐

(e) Can be safely treated with oral steroids if topical treatments are difficult to administer ☐ ☐

3.5 Healing chronic wounds

(a) The management of chronic wounds currently costs the NHS about £1 billion a year ☐ ☐

(b) Compression bandages are effective in arterial leg ulcers ☐ ☐

(c) Systemic factors (eg. renal disease) can impair healing ☐ ☐

(d) Fibroblasts play little part in the healing process ☐ ☐

(e) Bioengineered skin products are effective treatment ☐ ☐

3.6 Skin scarring

(a) Occurs because of injury to the epidermis ☐ ☐

(b) Is often a permanent consequence of accidents in children ☐ ☐

(c) Scars usually take less than six months to pale and mature ☐ ☐

(d) Scars can now be made to disappear ☐ ☐

(e) If keloid, scars are best treated by simple surgical excision ☐ ☐

3.7 Skin cancer

T   F

(a) The incidence of melanoma has doubled over the last twenty years ☐ ☐

(b) Most cannot be attributed to excessive exposure to the sun ☐ ☐

(c) Sunscreens with a high protection factor always prevent sunburn ☐ ☐

(d) Sun beds are a source of intensive exposure to infrared radiation ☐ ☐

(e) For prevention, using sunscreens is more important than measures to avoid exposure to the sun ☐ ☐

3.8 Scalp ringworm

(a) Is common in inner city children in the United Kingdom ☐ ☐

(b) Cannot be spread from person to person ☐ ☐

(c) Is easy to diagnose because of the well defined clinical presentation ☐ ☐

(d) Mycological analysis is advisable before starting treatment ☐ ☐

(e) Can be cleared with antifungal shampoos ☐ ☐

3.9 Herpes zoster

(a) Has an equal incidence in all age groups after the age of thirty ☐ ☐

(b) Can occur during chemotherapy or radiotherapy for malignancy ☐ ☐

(c) Is associated with pain which usually follows the appearance of the blisters ☐ ☐

(d) Antiviral treatment significantly reduces the risk of prolonged pain ☐ ☐

(e) Tricyclic antidepressants or gabapentin can be used for treating postherpetic neuralgia ☐ ☐

3.10 Iron deficiency anaemia

(a) Is most commonly caused in men by blood loss from the gastrointestinal tract ☐ ☐

T   F

(b) Is a known consequence of regular aspirin use ☐ ☐

(c) Has a different pathological basis from anaemia associated with chronic diseases ☐ ☐

(d) Is a cardinal sign of gastrointestinal cancer ☐ ☐

(e) Can be attributed to a poor diet based on history alone ☐ ☐

☐ ☐

3.11 Acute myeloid leukaemia

(a) Is more common in children than adults ☐ ☐

(b) Is an abnormality of the cell line that forms neutrophils and monocytes ☐ ☐

(c) Frequently presents with evidence of a bleeding tendency ☐ ☐

(d) Is associated with exposure to irradiation ☐ ☐

(e) Has a poorer prognosis in patients aged less than sixty ☐ ☐

3.12 Treatment of cutaneous ulcers

(a) Diuretics are more effective than pressure bandaging for venous ulceration ☐ ☐

(b) Support tights are useful for atherosclerotic ulcers ☐ ☐

(c) Benzoyl peroxide 20% should be avoided if the ulcer is infected ☐ ☐

(d) Gravitational dermatitis may be due to neomycin or lanolin sensitivity ☐ ☐

(e) Ciprofloxacin is recommended if complicated by *Pseudomonas* infection ☐ ☐

3.13 *Granuloma annulare*

(a) May occur at any age including young children ☐ ☐

(b) May respond to intra-lesional triamcinolone injections ☐ ☐

T   F

(c) In more than 50% of cases is associated with diabetes mellitus ☐ ☐

(d) Seldom resolves spontaneously ☐ ☐

(e) Classically occurs over the knuckles ☐ ☐

3.14 Erythema nodosum is associated with

(a) Streptococcal infection ☐ ☐

(b) Erythromycin ☐ ☐

(c) Tuberculosis ☐ ☐

(d) Crohn's disease ☐ ☐

(e) Cat scratch fever ☐ ☐

3.15 Tinea capitis

(a) The incidence has decreased in recent years ☐ ☐

(b) The diagnosis can be reliably made using Woods light ☐ ☐

(c) Shampoo treatments are licensed for treating children ☐ ☐

(d) Papules sometimes occur on the ears as the condition is treated ☐ ☐

(e) The boggy swelling of a kerion is due to inflammation ☐ ☐

3.16 Chickenpox infection

(a) Is characterised by a rash which first appears on the extremities ☐ ☐

(b) Is spread by the respiratory route ☐ ☐

(c) Is complicated by Reye's syndrome ☐ ☐

(d) Results in virus remaining latent in the peripheral nerve endings ☐ ☐

(e) Carries a high mortality for the neonate if contracted by the mother in the perinatal period ☐ ☐

Section 4

Circulation

4.1 In people over seventy

		T	F

a) Statins decrease the risk of stroke and major coronary events ☐ ☐

b) Diuretics are ineffective as first line treatment of hypertension ☐ ☐

c) Specialist units for CVA rehabilitation are effective in decreasing the risk of long-term institutional care, dependency, and death ☐ ☐

d) Calcium and vitamin D decreases the risk of non-vertebral fractures in healthy over sixty-five-year-olds ☐ ☐

e) Cholinesterase inhibitors produce major improvements in cognition and behaviour in demented patients ☐ ☐

4.2 In heart disease

a) There is a clear threshold that separates hypertensive patients who will experience future cardiovascular events from those who will not ☐ ☐

b) Left ventricular hypertrophy with hypertension is a significant risk factor ☐ ☐

c) Sedentary lifestyle is a risk factor in men ☐ ☐

d) Mathematical models are poor at predicting risk ☐ ☐

e) Obesity is a more potent risk factor in women than in men ☐ ☐

4.3 Deep venous thrombosis

a) Is common after major abdominal surgery ☐ ☐

b) Can be mimicked by a ruptured Baker's cyst ☐ ☐

c) One in twenty is complicated by potentially fatal pulmonary emboli before treatment ☐ ☐

T   F

d)   Is less common after ischaemic stroke than after myocardial infarction

e)   Perioperative antithrombotic prophylaxis is safe and effective

4.4 Stroke

a)   Most are ischaemic rather than haemorrhagic

b)   The incidence is lower in Afro-Caribbeans

c)   The number is increasing, despite effective treatment for hypertension

d)   Old age, diabetes and tobacco smoking are minor risk factors

e)   Aspirin is the key to treatment of haemorrhagic stroke

4.5 Stroke

a)   Is the second leading cause of death in the world

b)   Primary prevention is ineffective

c)   Antiplatelet drugs are effective in secondary prevention

d)   The absolute risk is greatest at blood pressures that would not currently be treated with drugs

e)   Angiotensin converting enzyme inhibitors can reduce stroke in high risk patients with normal blood pressure

4.6 Atrial fibrillation

a)   Is the most common sustained disorder of cardiac rhythm

b)   The risk of stroke is the same whether AF is persistent or paroxysmal

c)   Warfarin decreases the incidence of stroke by over 90%

d)   The numbers of patients needed to treat are greater for primary prevention than for secondary prevention of stroke

T   F

e)   Aspirin is as effective as warfarin in preventing stroke   ☐ ☐

4.7 Antithrombolytic therapy

a)   Aspirin inhibits cyclo-oxygenase, the rate limiting step in thromboxane A2 synthesis   ☐ ☐

b)   Aspirin can be used safely in patients with thrombocytopaenia   ☐ ☐

c)   Dipyridamole has a long lasting effect on phosphodiesterase   ☐ ☐

d)   Warfarin inhibits clotting factors that are dependent on vitamin K   ☐ ☐

e)   Warfarin metabolism is inhibited by cimetidine   ☐ ☐

4.8 Chronic heart failure

a)   Requires a diuretic and ACE inhibitor as preferred first line treatment   ☐ ☐

b)   Spironolactone is an outdated form of treatment   ☐ ☐

c)   Beta-blockers are absolutely contraindicated   ☐ ☐

d)   Non-steroidal anti-inflammatory drugs can worsen symptoms   ☐ ☐

e)   Around 10% of new cases are primarily due to valve disease   ☐ ☐

4.9 Newly diagnosed hypertension

a)   Has a secondary cause in 25% of patients   ☐ ☐

b)   May be reversible if lifestyle changes are adhered to   ☐ ☐

c)   An ECG is no longer needed as part of the work up   ☐ ☐

d)   Family history is unimportant   ☐ ☐

e)   With severe diastolic hypertension (115–129 mmHg) the number needed to treat to prevent death, stroke and myocardial infarction is as low as three   ☐ ☐

4.10 Hypertension

		T	F
a)	Doxazosin treatment is associated with congestive cardiac failure	☐	☐
b)	Chlorthalidone, amlodipine, and lisinopril are equally effective	☐	☐
c)	Thiazide diuretics are the least effective drugs for preventing stroke	☐	☐
d)	Most patients require two or more drugs to control their blood pressure to less than 140/90	☐	☐
e)	Blood pressure control is easier in older patients because of better compliance	☐	☐

4.11 ECGs

a)	Hyperkalaemia is associated with flat T waves	☐	☐
b)	Hypokalaemia prolongs the QT interval	☐	☐
c)	Hypothermia causes J waves	☐	☐
d)	Hypothyroidism causes tachycardia	☐	☐
e)	Hypercalcaemia is associated with a long QT interval	☐	☐

4.12 Exercise tolerance testing

a)	ST segment depression is the most reliable indicator for exercise-induced ischaemia	☐	☐
b)	In men under thirty and women under forty, a positive test is more likely to be a false positive than a true positive	☐	☐
c)	Has the greatest diagnostic value in patients with an intermediate risk of ischaemic heart disease	☐	☐
d)	A complete test takes twenty-one minutes with seven stages of 3 minutes	☐	☐
e)	Can be done within a week of a myocardial infarction	☐	☐

4.13 Myocardial ischaemia

a)	Changes in the ST segment and T waves are specific	☐	☐

T   F

b) The ECG can be normal in patients with severe and widespread coronary artery disease □ □

c) In patients presenting to hospital with acute myocardial infarction, more than 80% will have typical and diagnostic ECG changes in their initial trace □ □

d) Atrial fibrillation is the most common supraventricular arrhythmia after MI □ □

e) Suppression of ventricular ectopics by antiarrhythmic drugs prevents subsequent ventricular fibrillation □ □

4.14 Sinus tachycardia

a) Usually exceeds 200 beats per minute in adults □ □

b) P waves have abnormal morphology □ □

c) The ventricular rhythm is irregular □ □

d) The atrial rate is the same as the ventricular rate □ □

e) In the absence of an obvious underlying cause, should prompt consideration of atrial flutter or atrial tachycardia □ □

4.15 Causes of bradycardia include

a) Hyperthermia □ □

b) Hyperthyroidism □ □

c) Sick sinus syndrome □ □

d) Raised intracranial pressure □ □

e) Inferior myocardial infarction □ □

4.16 Anticoagulant therapy

a) Antidepressants can enhance the anticoagulant effect □ □

T   F

b)   Oral contraceptives increase the effects of anticoagulants   ☐ ☐

c)   In congestive cardiac failure, the dose of warfarin is higher than normal   ☐ ☐

d)   The risk of bleeding increases substantially when the INR is greater than five   ☐ ☐

e)   Older patients generally need higher doses of warfarin   ☐ ☐

4.17 Peripheral arterial disease

a)   Can usually be diagnosed on the basis of the history   ☐ ☐

b)   The risk to the limb is high, but the risk to life is low   ☐ ☐

c)   Is rarely associated with diabetes mellitus   ☐ ☐

d)   Treatment with a statin is not indicated unless the patient has angina as well   ☐ ☐

e)   Surgery is only of benefit when the femoral pulses are normal   ☐ ☐

4.18 Acute myocardial infarction

a)   Shows an abnormal ECG in less than 50% of patients in the early stages   ☐ ☐

b)   Typically is diagnosed by elevated ST segments in two or more anatomically distant leads   ☐ ☐

c)   Is significantly more likely in a non-smoking obese man of forty-five, than a smoking woman with a normal BMI aged sixty-five   ☐ ☐

d)   Is more likely to be complicated by supraventricular than ventricular arrhythmias in the first twenty-four hours post infarction   ☐ ☐

e)   Warrants antithrombolytic therapy on enzyme changes in absence of ECG changes   ☐ ☐

4.19 Physiological measurements regarded as within the normal range include

T F

a) A regular heart rate anywhere in the range 60–99 beats/min ☐ ☐

b) Upright P waves in leads I and II of an ECG ☐ ☐

c) A core (rectal) temperature of 35°C ☐ ☐

d) Systolic BP < 90 ☐ ☐

e) Diastolic BP < 90 ☐ ☐

4.20 The calcium channel blocker nifedipine

a) Has a useful therapeutic anti-arrhythmic effect ☐ ☐

b) Should not be used with beta-blockers ☐ ☐

c) Is particularly valuable in the first month after myocardial infarction ☐ ☐

d) May cause ischaemic cardiac pain within half-an-hour of starting the drug ☐ ☐

e) May be used to manage Raynaud's phenomenon ☐ ☐

4.21 In patients with infective endocarditis

a) Mortality is greater if the infecting organism is Streptococcus viridans, than if it is fungal ☐ ☐

b) Echocardiography plays a key role in assessing prognosis ☐ ☐

c) The disease rarely presents in an occult fashion ☐ ☐

d) Blood cultures are persistently negative in 5–10% ☐ ☐

e) Sudden mitral regurgitation may occur ☐ ☐

Section 5

Respiration

		T	F

5.1 In asthma

a) Decreased diurnal variation of peak flow is diagnostic ☐ ☐

b) The prevalence is about 10% of the population ☐ ☐

c) Most sufferers are atopic ☐ ☐

d) Hospital admission for asthma is associated with a higher risk of death from asthma ☐ ☐

e) Intermittent corticosteroids are given at step FIVE of the BTS guidelines ☐ ☐

5.2 In chronic obstructive pulmonary disease (COPD)

a) Inhaled corticosteroids prevent the progressive decline in lung function ☐ ☐

b) Lung surgery is of little benefit in emphysema ☐ ☐

c) Physical exercise can improve quality of life ☐ ☐

d) Stopping smoking is of marginal benefit ☐ ☐

e) Leukotriene antagonists are a significant breakthrough in treatment ☐ ☐

5.3 Community acquired pneumonia in adults

a) Accurate diagnosis is straightforward ☐ ☐

b) A low respiratory rate is one of the most important indicators of disease severity ☐ ☐

c) Atypical organisms (eg. mycoplasma and chlamydia) are uncommon ☐ ☐

d) In the elderly, confusion is not a common feature ☐ ☐

T   F

e) Management is based on sound evidence from randomised controlled trials ☐ ☐

5.4 Asthma in children

a) Is rare under the age of five ☐ ☐

b) Is commonly associated with a family history of asthma or eczema ☐ ☐

c) Is typically associated with inspiratory stridor ☐ ☐

d) Recent use of salbutamol is typically associated with an increased pulse rate ☐ ☐

e) Is usually confirmed by measuring peak flow variability in the pre-school child ☐ ☐

5.5 Respiratory failure

a) In the UK is most commonly caused by an acute relapse of infection in chronic bronchitis and emphysema ☐ ☐

b) Is a complication of poliomyelitis ☐ ☐

c) Can be precipitated by postoperative sedation in patients with COPD ☐ ☐

d) Is treated initially with 28% oxygen ☐ ☐

e) Rarely achieves significant improvement by removal of secretions ☐ ☐

5.6 In the treatment of asthma with salbutamol

a) Salbutamol is a selective ß2–adrenoreceptor stimulant with a duration of action of about four hours ☐ ☐

b) One aerosol container delivers 200 doses ☐ ☐

c) Side–effects include hyperkalaemia after intravenous administration ☐ ☐

d) Is best given by subcutaneous or intravenous route for severe acute asthma ☐ ☐

T   F

e) Should be avoided in patients with bronchospasm and co-existing cardiac disease ☐ ☐

5.7 Respiratory function tests used in the assessment of airflow limitation

a) The peak expiratory flow rate (PEFR) is measured with a Wright meter and the average of three test results is recorded ☐ ☐

b) The PEFR is defined as the fastest flow rate sustained for ten millisecs ☐ ☐

c) The PEFR is a good measure of airflow limitation but intra-subject reliability is poor ☐ ☐

d) With a Vitalograph spirometer the FEV1, expressed as a percentage of FVC is an excellent measure of airflow limitation ☐ ☐

e) With restrictive lung disease the FEV1 and the FVC are reduced in the same proportion ☐ ☐

5.8 Legionnaire's disease

a) Affects men and women equally ☐ ☐

b) May present with abdominal symptoms ☐ ☐

c) Has an increased incidence in patients on dialysis ☐ ☐

d) Has an incubation period of fourteen to twenty-one days ☐ ☐

e) Is optimally treated with oral tetracycline ☐ ☐

5.9 In patients with chronic obstructive pulmonary disease

a) If aged under forty years, alpha-1 anti-trypsin deficiency should be considered ☐ ☐

b) Bullae seen on chest X-ray are pathognomonic ☐ ☐

c) Airflow limitation as measured by FEV1 can never be reversed to normal values ☐ ☐

T   F

d)   The FEV1 is reduced by 70% in lung function tests by definition   ☐ ☐

e)   Vaccination against influenza is recommended   ☐ ☐

5.10 The following are recognised causes of drug-induced asthma

a)   Ibuprofen   ☐ ☐

b)   Calcium channel-blockers   ☐ ☐

c)   Paracetamol   ☐ ☐

d)   Cardio-selective beta-blockers   ☐ ☐

e)   Propellants used in salbutamol metered-dose inhalers   ☐ ☐

5.11 Mycoplasma

a)   Infections are best treated with metronidazole or flucytosine   ☐ ☐

b)   May be found in endoscope-washer/disinfectors   ☐ ☐

c)   Treatment regimes should be initiated only after liver function tests have been performed   ☐ ☐

d)   Are intracellular pathogens which cause a host response of granuloma formation   ☐ ☐

e)   Commonly causes disseminated disease in patients with AIDS   ☐ ☐

5.12 Tuberculosis

a)   Is the single biggest infectious disease globally   ☐ ☐

b)   The incidence has been static in the United Kingdom over the last ten years   ☐ ☐

c)   Is associated with drug dependence   ☐ ☐

d)   Resistance to antibacterial agents is becoming less common   ☐ ☐

T   F

e) Is prevented by BCG, which is a heat-killed strain of Mycobacterium bovis ☐ ☐

5.13 Haemoptysis

a) Is a rare symptom of bronchial carcinoma ☐ ☐

b) Can be caused by epistaxis ☐ ☐

c) Is a symptom of acute left ventricular failure ☐ ☐

d) Is a complication of treatment with warfarin ☐ ☐

e) Should always be investigated with a chest X-ray ☐ ☐

5.14 Causes of solitary pulmonary nodules include

a) Metastasis from renal carcinoma ☐ ☐

b) Asbestosis ☐ ☐

c) Carcinoid ☐ ☐

d) Rheumatoid lung disease ☐ ☐

e) Sarcoidosis ☐ ☐

5.15 Domiciliary oxygen therapy

a) Is indicated in COPD if the FEV1<1.5 litres, the FVC<2.0 litres, and arterial oxygen tension is <7.3kPa and CO2>6 kPa over at least a three-week period ☐ ☐

b) Has to be used for over 20 hours a day to be of benefit ☐ ☐

c) Can reduce mortality in severe COPD ☐ ☐

d) Can only be prescribed after recommendation from a hospital consultant ☐ ☐

e) Enables patients to maintain self-control over their lives ☐ ☐

5.16 The following are occupational lung diseases   T   F

a)   Asthma

b)   Mesothelioma

c)   Pneumoconiosis

d)   Benign pleural disease

e)   Allergic alveolitis

5.17 In lower respiratory tract illness in adults in primary care

a)   Nearly three out of four patients are prescribed an antibiotic

b)   A minority have abnormal physical signs

c)   Discoloured sputum is associated with higher morbidity

d)   Regardless of treatment, the cough lasts for two to three weeks

e)   Patient satisfaction is reduced if antibiotics are not prescribed

5.18 Acute cough in pre-school children

a)   Two out of three visit their GP at least annually for an acute respiratory infection, the majority with a cough

b)   Costs the NHS about £20 million a year

c)   One in four are no better after two weeks

d)   Under 50% are prescribed an antibiotic in the UK

e)   About 10% experience one or more complications

5.19 Hoarseness

a)   Is associated with hyperthyroidism

b)   Needs referral to an ENT specialist only if it lasts longer than twelve weeks

		T	F
c)	Is an occupational hazard of professional singers	☐	☐
d)	Can be caused by gastro-oesophageal reflux disease (GORD)	☐	☐
e)	Is a symptom of tracheitis	☐	☐

5.20 Acute (over minutes or hours) dyspnoea is caused by

a)	Pneumothorax	☐	☐
b)	Pulmonary embolism	☐	☐
c)	Anaemia	☐	☐
d)	Pleural effusion	☐	☐
e)	Sarcoidosis	☐	☐

Section 6

Homeostasis and hormones

6.1 Treating benign prostatic hypertrophy

            T   F

(a) Alpha-blockers are effective

(b) 5 alpha reductase inhibitors are ineffective

(c) Transurethral resection of the prostate gland (TURP) has been superseded by less invasive surgical procedures

(d) Rye grass pollen extract can have some benefit

(e) Retrograde ejaculation is common after TURP

6.2 Hypokalaemia

(a) Is a known side-effect of treatment with digoxin

(b) Can cause cardiac arrest

(c) Typically presents with hypotension and tiredness

(d) Is one presenting feature of chronic laxative abuse

(e) Can be an artefact of venesection when an IV infusion is present in the same arm

6.3 Apoptosis

(a) Is promoted by tumour necrosis factor

(b) Is inhibited by TSH

(c) High levels in breast tumours seem to predict better survival

(d) Plays a part in Alzheimer's disease and other adult neurodegenerative disorders

	T	F
(e) Has no role in inflammatory conditions and autoimmune disorders	☐	☐

6.4 Chronic fatigue

	T	F
(a) Is associated with desynchronisation of circadian rhythms	☐	☐
(b) Is rarely precipitated by stressful life events	☐	☐
(c) Illness beliefs may perpetuate the condition	☐	☐
(d) Can be effectively treated with cognitive behaviour therapy	☐	☐
(e) Patient education to encourage graded exercise is ineffective	☐	☐

6.5 Testicular cancer

	T	F
(a) Is the most common cancer in young men	☐	☐
(b) Has an incidence which is decreasing	☐	☐
(c) Cure rates can exceed 95%	☐	☐
(d) Is not associated with testicular maldescent	☐	☐
(e) Is one of the cancers which has a familial risk	☐	☐

6.6 Reye's syndrome

	T	F
(a) Is caused by a failure of mitochondria	☐	☐
(b) Is usually associated with paracetamol use in young children with fever	☐	☐
(c) Is increasing in incidence	☐	☐
(d) Does not occur over the age of twelve	☐	☐
(e) Can cause encephalopathy, hepatic abnormality, and metabolic decompensation	☐	☐

6.7 Cancers of the head and neck   T   F

(a) There is an association with chewing betel or araca nuts   ☐ ☐

(b) Squamous cell cancers are one of the most common cancers world-wide   ☐ ☐

(c) They are more common in women than men   ☐ ☐

(d) Pain in the ears is an uncommon presenting symptom   ☐ ☐

(e) The prognosis is poor because most patients present with distant metastases   ☐ ☐

6.8 Management of renal colic in general practice

(a) The condition is more common in men than in women   ☐ ☐

(b) Intramuscular diclofenac 75 mg is effective first line management for pain   ☐ ☐

(c) If severe pain does not remit within twenty-four hours the patient should be admitted to hospital   ☐ ☐

(d) Hospital investigation is not indicated after a single attack if it settles at home   ☐ ☐

(e) The presence of haematuria does not support the diagnosis   ☐ ☐

6.9 Urinary incontinence in women

(a) It is reported by 14% of women   ☐ ☐

(b) Physiotherapy is ineffective   ☐ ☐

(c) Systematic reviews show that colposuspension has cure rates of up to 90%   ☐ ☐

(d) It is rarely associated with urinary infection   ☐ ☐

(e) Stress incontinence is the most common form   ☐ ☐

6.10 Chronic renal disease   T   F

(a)   Significant renal dysfunction can be present when serum creatinine is
      normal or only slightly abnormal   ☐   ☐

(b)   Symptoms of renal failure occur early in the disease   ☐   ☐

(c)   Cardiovascular disease accounts for very few deaths   ☐   ☐

(d)   Anaemia is a late complication   ☐   ☐

(e)   Blood pressure control of 160/95 or less is acceptable   ☐   ☐

6.11 Renal transplantation

(a)   Was first done successfully in the early 1950s   ☐   ☐

(b)   Survival rates from living donors can exceed 10 years   ☐   ☐

(c)   Improved road safety has led to fewer donor organs being available ☐   ☐

(d)   The incidence of renal failure is static   ☐   ☐

(e)   Most patients die from renal failure   ☐   ☐

6.12 Metformin treatment in diabetes mellitus

(a)   Is indicated if the patient is underweight   ☐   ☐

(b)   Can reduce cardiovascular risk   ☐   ☐

(c)   Is contraindicated in patients with mild renal impairment   ☐   ☐

(d)   Needs to be withdrawn before general anaesthesia   ☐   ☐

(e)   Should be continued during an admission for myocardial infarction ☐   ☐

6.13 Managing thyroid dysfunction

(a)   Hypothyroidism may exist with normal concentrations of thyroxine
      and TSH   ☐   ☐

(b)   The pituitary thyrotroph cells are highly sensitive to minor changes
      in thyroid hormone concentrations   ☐   ☐

T F

(c) Patients with a raised TSH and normal thyroxine level generally benefit from early use of thyroxine replacement therapy ☐ ☐

(d) TSH levels can be normal in profound hypothyroidism secondary to pituitary or hypothalamic disease ☐ ☐

(e) The presence of anti-thyroid peroxidase antibodies with a raised TSH is an indication for early treatment with thyroxine ☐ ☐

6.14 Using tumour markers for screening or monitoring disease

(a) CEA is specific for colorectal carcinoma ☐ ☐

(b) Serum levels of CA125 are elevated in both ovarian and pancreatic carcinoma ☐ ☐

(c) AFP is likely to be of little prognostic value in the management of testicular teratoma ☐ ☐

(d) A rise of HCG in pregnancy is diagnostic of choriocarcinoma ☐ ☐

(e) A PSA of 8 ng/ml implies extracapsular spread of prostatic carcinoma ☐ ☐

6.15 Managing uncomplicated urinary tract infections

(a) Over 50% of patients will be asymptomatic at three days without antibiotics ☐ ☐

(b) Cranberry juice has been shown to give symptomatic relief ☐ ☐

(c) The presence of both protein and nitrites on diagnostic stick testing of urine is a reliable indication of infection ☐ ☐

(d) The risk of pyelonephritis is sufficient to justify treating all patients with antibiotics ☐ ☐

(e) A three-day course of antibiotic treatment will relieve symptoms in 88% of patients ☐ ☐

Section 7

The 'Senses'

7.1 Treatment of migraine

		T	F
(a)	Triptans are effective but can cause headache	☐	☐
(b)	Beta-blockers are used for attack therapy	☐	☐
(c)	Lisinopril has a clinically important prophylactic effect	☐	☐
(d)	NSAIDs show some prophylactic effect, as well as giving relief in the acute attack	☐	☐
(e)	Sodium valproate has no preventive effect	☐	☐

7.2 Cataract surgery

a)	The benefits and risks in the very elderly are less clear	☐	☐
b)	Increasing age is associated with poorer outcomes	☐	☐
c)	Associated age-related maculopathy does not affect outcome	☐	☐
d)	Cardiovascular disease carries higher risks during surgery	☐	☐
e)	Is usually performed under general anaesthetic	☐	☐

7.3 Otitis media in children

a)	Antibiotics are of marginal benefit	☐	☐
b)	Most children receive antibiotics	☐	☐
c)	A wait and see strategy is feasible and acceptable to parents for children who are not very unwell	☐	☐
d)	Antibiotics cause diarrhoea in 50%	☐	☐

T   F

e) The main benefit of antibiotics occurs after the first 24 hours when symptoms are resolving ☐ ☐

7.4 Headache

a) Can be caused by medication overuse ☐ ☐

b) Migraine, tension headache and cluster headache account for the type of headache in less than half of consulting patients ☐ ☐

c) Migraine causes more disability than epilepsy ☐ ☐

d) Can be a presenting feature of glaucoma ☐ ☐

e) Subacute carbon monoxide poisoning should be considered ☐ ☐

7.5 Chronic suppurative otitis media

a) Can be confused with otitis externa ☐ ☐

b) The discharge comes through a perforation in the tympanic membrane ☐ ☐

c) Cholesteatoma is a potential complication ☐ ☐

d) Topical antibiotics are less effective in acute treatment than oral ones ☐ ☐

e) Can lead to erosion of the ossicles ☐ ☐

7.6 Myopia

a) The prevalence of visual impairment caused by myopia is decreasing ☐ ☐

b) A large part of peoples' refractive status is genetically determined ☐ ☐

c) Visual experiences early in life can affect ocular growth and eventual refractive status ☐ ☐

d) Is often associated with glaucoma ☐ ☐

e) The image is focused in front of the retina ☐ ☐

7.7 Age-related macular degeneration   T   F

a) The main symptom of the non-exudative form is gradual increase in difficulty in seeing fine detail ☐ ☐

b) The main symptom of the exudative form is central blurring of gradual onset ☐ ☐

c) Tunnel vision is a late feature ☐ ☐

d) Men are significantly more likely than women to suffer from the exudative form ☐ ☐

e) Thermal laser treatment can restore vision that has been lost ☐ ☐

7.8 Acute otitis media in a one-year-old

(a) Is seldom associated with prolonged deafness ☐ ☐

(b) Is usually accompanied by profuse discharge ☐ ☐

(c) Should be treated with a ten-day course of an antibiotic ☐ ☐

(d) Commonly starts with similar signs to those of early meningitis ☐ ☐

(e) Will typically be associated with tonsillitis ☐ ☐

7.9 Hoarseness of the voice can be a presenting sign of

(a) Developing laryngeal oedema ☐ ☐

(b) Hyperthyroidism ☐ ☐

(c) Cancer of the tongue ☐ ☐

(d) Hysterical conversion syndrome ☐ ☐

(e) Nicotine dependence ☐ ☐

7.10 Double vision as a presenting symptom may be due to

(a) A cataract causing a double image in one eye ☐ ☐

(b) Temporal arteritis ☐ ☐

	T	F

(c) Cavernous sinus thrombosis ☐ ☐

(d) Fourth cranial nerve infarction ☐ ☐

(e) A problem of the sixth cranial nerve if the diplopia is predominantly vertical ☐ ☐

7.11 Vertigo

(a) Is defined as a sense of general unsteadiness when standing ☐ ☐

(b) Is associated with progressive deafness in Menière's disease ☐ ☐

(c) Is treated with stelazine as the drug of choice ☐ ☐

(d) Is a common symptom of viral labyrinthitis ☐ ☐

(e) May be treated by recurrent repositioning of the head (Epley's manoeuvre) ☐ ☐

7.12 Dysphonia

(a) In 60% of cases have had antibiotics before being referred ☐ ☐

(b) Interpersonal difficulties are three times as common in patients with functional dysphonia ☐ ☐

(c) In functional dysphonia, education is less helpful than speech therapy ☐ ☐

(d) Is associated with gastro-oesophageal reflux ☐ ☐

(e) Prescribing rest for vocal hyperfunction is often effective ☐ ☐

7.13 Migraine

(a) Ergotamine will relieve most attacks ☐ ☐

(b) The majority of attacks are of the 'classical' type ☐ ☐

(c) Horner's syndrome is associated with cluster migraine ☐ ☐

(d) Sodium valproate has been shown to be of little use prophylactically ☐ ☐

T F

(e) 5HT receptor blockers (Triptans) should not be given in patients on cimetidine ☐ ☐

7.14 The condition of acute epiglottitis in children

(a) Is associated with a Haemophilus influenzae septicaemia ☐ ☐

(b) Usually occurs in children under two years ☐ ☐

(c) Should be treated with intravenous cefotaxime ☐ ☐

(d) Characteristically causes the child to prefer to lie prone ☐ ☐

(e) Is characterised by stridor that worsens as the child deteriorates ☐ ☐

7.15 Risk factors for hearing loss include

(a) Otitis media with effusion (Glue ear) ☐ ☐

(b) Meningitis ☐ ☐

(c) Down's syndrome ☐ ☐

(d) Tetracycline treatment ☐ ☐

(e) Barotrauma ☐ ☐

Section 8

Digestion and nutrition

8.1 Jaundice

		T	F
a)	Can be caused by oestrogens	☐	☐
b)	Occupation is of little relevance	☐	☐
c)	Is associated with blue nails	☐	☐
d)	Is most commonly prehepatic in nature	☐	☐
e)	3% of the population have raised bilirubin (Gilbert's syndrome)	☐	☐

8.2 Obesity in childhood

a)	Advice to overweight children should be to maintain current weight or gain weight slowly rather than lose weight	☐	☐
b)	Restricting the diet is better than healthy eating habits	☐	☐
c)	Is associated with psychosocial problems	☐	☐
d)	Progression to adult obesity is inevitable	☐	☐
e)	Is commonly associated with parental obesity	☐	☐

8.3 Acute dysphagia

a)	Can be caused by stroke	☐	☐
b)	Radiology is less rewarding than endoscopy in clarifying the cause of upper oesophageal causes of dysphagia	☐	☐
c)	With solids and liquids, in the absence of weight loss, is likely to be caused by achalasia	☐	☐
d)	Motility disturbances of the oesophagus are rare	☐	☐

T   F

e)   Alendroic acid can cause oesophageal strictures   ☐   ☐

8.4 Gastric cancer

a)   Helicobacter pylori infection is not a risk factor   ☐   ☐

b)   Pernicious anaemia is a risk factor   ☐   ☐

c)   It can present with iron deficiency anaemia   ☐   ☐

d)   It is incurable in about half of patients at presentation   ☐   ☐

e)   Dysphagia is not a feature   ☐   ☐

8.5 Dyspepsia

a)   Frequent heartburn is a cardinal symptom of gastrointestinal reflux   ☐   ☐

b)   Classic ulcer symptoms do not occur in functional dyspepsia   ☐   ☐

c)   Can be confused with angina pectoris   ☐   ☐

d)   Is rarely linked with possibility of cancer by patients   ☐   ☐

e)   Alarm symptoms include anorexia and weight loss   ☐   ☐

8.6 Ascites

a)   Is associated with portal hypertension   ☐   ☐

b)   Rare causes include myxoedema   ☐   ☐

c)   Hyperalbuminaemia is a common finding   ☐   ☐

d)   If minimal, cannot be confirmed by ultrasound   ☐   ☐

e)   Most patients respond to dietary sodium restriction and diuretics   ☐   ☐

8.7 Abnormal liver function tests in primary care

a)   Are usually adequately investigated   ☐   ☐

T F

b)   Offer an important chance to identify treatable chronic liver disease ☐ ☐

c)   Are commonly caused by alcoholic liver disease ☐ ☐

d)   Often revert to normal when repeated ☐ ☐

e)   Can be caused by minor viral illness ☐ ☐

8.8 Obesity in adults

a)   Is defined as a BMI of equal or more than 30 ☐ ☐

b)   Surgical intervention is ineffective in morbid obesity ☐ ☐

c)   The prevalence is increasing ☐ ☐

d)   Reductions of 500–1000 kcal a day are needed to produce weight loss
      at the rate of 0.45 to 0.90 kg per week ☐ ☐

e)   Appetite suppressants should be regarded as the last resort ☐ ☐

8.9 In gastro-oesophageal reflux disease (GORD)

a)   Heartburn affects over a third of the population at some time each
      month ☐ ☐

b)   More than two thirds of heartburn sufferers progress to chronic
      symptoms ☐ ☐

c)   Relief of heartburn predicts healing of oesophagitis ☐ ☐

d)   All patients on proton pump inhibitors for GORD should have
      Helicobacter pylori eradicated ☐ ☐

e)   Onset over the age of thirty-five should be investigated by endoscopy ☐ ☐

8.10 In functional gastro-intestinal disorders

a)   Treatment with tricylic antidepressants is effective even in the
      absence of depression ☐ ☐

b)   Irritable bowel syndrome is the least common disorder ☐ ☐

T   F

c) Women attending gastroenterology clinics often have a history of sexual and emotional abuse ☐ ☐

d) In patients who are resistant to treatment, the incidence of emotional distress is higher in general practice than in hospital outpatients ☐ ☐

e) There is unequivocal evidence that psychological treatments are effective ☐ ☐

8.11 Nutrition

a) Up to a third of cancers might be prevented by a healthy diet ☐ ☐

b) Genetic make-up has no direct consequences for nutrition ☐ ☐

c) Glucosamine is unlikely to be of benefit in osteoarthritis ☐ ☐

d) Folic acid before conception can protect against neural tube defects ☐ ☐

e) Moderate to low alcohol intake is associated with a reduced risk of heart disease but an increased risk of cancer ☐ ☐

8.12 Carcinoma of the oesophagus

a) Is commoner in women than in men ☐ ☐

b) Has an overall survival rate five years after surgical resection of 30–40% ☐ ☐

c) Is strongly related to both tobacco and alcohol use ☐ ☐

d) Usually presents early with retrosternal pain ☐ ☐

e) Is associated with Barrett's oesophagus ☐ ☐

8.13 Giardiasis

a) Is unlikely if travellers stay in good quality hotels ☐ ☐

b) Is treated with ciprofloxacin as the treatment of choice ☐ ☐

c) Is the main parasitic cause of travellers' diarrhoea ☐ ☐

		T	F

d) May produce a malabsorption or sprue-like syndrome ☐ ☐

e) In most carriers will be symptomatic ☐ ☐

8.14 In infantile gastroenteris

a) Oral antibiotics are useful if the child is being treated at home ☐ ☐

b) Rotavirus is the most common cause worldwide ☐ ☐

c) Infants in hospital should be barrier nursed ☐ ☐

d) A dry tongue is a late sign of dehydration ☐ ☐

e) Mothers should be advised to make up a simple rehydration mixture using sugar and salt ☐ ☐

8.15 In acute infectious hepatitis (type A)

a) There is general progression to cirrhosis after a number of years ☐ ☐

b) There is a contraindication to combined oral contraceptive pills ☐ ☐

c) Spread of virus is via faecal contamination ☐ ☐

d) Specific diagnostic signs can generally be recognised in blood films ☐ ☐

e) Good protection is afforded by adequate doses of prophylactic gamma globulin ☐ ☐

8.16 Dietary gluten enteropathy

a) Is exclusively a disorder of childhood ☐ ☐

b) May be associated with psoriasis ☐ ☐

c) Has a genetic basis with a familial pattern ☐ ☐

d) May be treated with gluten-free products, which can only be prescribed by a hospital specialist ☐ ☐

e) May predispose to small bowel lymphoma ☐ ☐

8.17 Chronic pancreatitis

T   F

a) Has a mean age of onset in Britain and Western Europe of about thirty-five years ☐ ☐

b) Is frequently associated with chronic duodenal ulceration ☐ ☐

c) Is a known concomitant of chronic alcoholism ☐ ☐

d) Is present with gallstones in more than 25% of patients ☐ ☐

e) May present with serous effusions of the pleural and peritoneal cavities ☐ ☐

8.18 Children with coeliac disease

a) Normally present with symptoms before they are two years old ☐ ☐

b) May become constipated ☐ ☐

c) Though losing weight, usually remain cheerful and active ☐ ☐

d) Gluten-free diet excludes all foods containing wheat, rye and barley ☐ ☐

e) On treatment, height and weight can be expected to return to normal centiles within three months ☐ ☐

8.19 Fissure-in-ano

a) The commonest site is mid-line posteriorly ☐ ☐

b) Is frequently associated with slight bleeding ☐ ☐

c) Pain is only present during defaecation ☐ ☐

d) Operative treatment is dilatation of the sphincter ☐ ☐

e) Is common, found in more than 10% of rectal complaints ☐ ☐

8.20 Trichinosis

a) Is predominantly found in India ☐ ☐

	T	F

b) The larval form of Trichinella spiralis is found in hares, pigs, dogs and cats ☐ ☐

c) Symptoms do not occur for twenty-one days ☐ ☐

d) The adult form in humans lodges in the intestine ☐ ☐

e) Myocardial and central nervous system involvement are rare ☐ ☐

8.21 Abdominal pain in a three-year-old may be due to

a) Tonsillitis ☐ ☐

b) Perthes disease ☐ ☐

c) Familial Mediterranean fever ☐ ☐

d) Helicobacter pylori infection ☐ ☐

e) Henoch Schonlein purpura ☐ ☐

8.22 Constipation is a side-effect of

a) Proton pump inhibitors ☐ ☐

b) Dextropropoxyphene ☐ ☐

c) Selective serotonin re-uptake inhibitors ☐ ☐

d) Dicyclomine hydrochloride ☐ ☐

e) Erythromycin ☐ ☐

Section 9

Reproduction

9.1 Sexually transmitted disease

		T	F
(a)	Cervical cancer is frequently associated with human papilloma virus type 16	☐	☐
(b)	A twenty-two-year-old man with a urethral discharge is more likely to be infected with Chlamydia trachomatis than gonorrhoea	☐	☐
(c)	Contact tracing is mandatory for cases of non-specific urethritis	☐	☐
(d)	Many genital herpes simplex infections are asymptomatic	☐	☐
(e)	Risk factors include unprotected oral sex	☐	☐

9.2 The 'combined' oral contraceptive pill

(a)	Increases the risk of haemolytic jaundice	☐	☐
(b)	Will put users at risk of pregnancy if taken concomitantly with a three-day course of penicillin V	☐	☐
(c)	Reduces blood levels of anti-thrombin III	☐	☐
(d)	Is associated with an increased incidence of carpal tunnel syndrome	☐	☐
(e)	Interacts with drug treatments for epilepsy	☐	☐

9.3 Considering AIDS

(a)	World-wide, heterosexual transmission is the dominant mode of spread	☐	☐
(b)	Weight loss of more than 10% of body weight is a major sign	☐	☐
(c)	There is an association with cryptococcal meningitis	☐	☐

T   F

(d) Antiretroviral treatment is available to the majority of people in developing countries ☐ ☐

(e) A raised CD4 count is associated with a worse prognosis ☐ ☐

9.4 Spontaneous first trimester miscarriage

(a) Does not require surgical evacuation after complete miscarriage ☐ ☐

(b) Cannot safely be managed in primary care ☐ ☐

(c) Should be managed medically rather than expectantly as it has few side-effects ☐ ☐

(d) Is commonly associated with infection and septicaemia ☐ ☐

(e) Can be confused with ectopic pregnancy ☐ ☐

9.5 Pelvic inflammatory disease

(a) Can be reliably diagnosed from clinical symptoms and signs ☐ ☐

(b) Is asymptomatic in the majority of cases ☐ ☐

(c) Is more common in those of African or Afro-Caribbean origin ☐ ☐

(d) Can be caused by infection with mycoplasma hominis ☐ ☐

(e) Can result in ectopic pregnancy in 10% of women who conceive ☐ ☐

9.6 The management of menorrhagia

(a) Women under forty should receive tranexamic acid before hospital referral ☐ ☐

(b) No woman should receive norethisterone as a first line treatment ☐ ☐

(c) Women should receive tranexamic acid or a NSAID as first line treatment ☐ ☐

(d) Endometrial cancer should be considered a common cause in women over forty ☐ ☐

	T	F

(e) Dilatation and curettage is the most effective surgical intervention ☐ ☐

9.7 Pre-eclamptic toxaemia

(a) Complicates more than 10% of pregnancies ☐ ☐

(b) Is associated with maternal death if severe ☐ ☐

(c) Is associated with under-production of prostacyclin and excessive production of thromboxane ☐ ☐

(d) Cannot be prevented with antiplatelet drugs ☐ ☐

(e) Is always accompanied by proteinuria ☐ ☐

9.8 In endometriosis

(a) A common symptom is pelvic pain ☐ ☐

(b) Diagnosis is easy from the patient's symptoms ☐ ☐

(c) First line management includes NSAID and the contraceptive pill ☐ ☐

(d) Referral is indicated where infertility is a problem ☐ ☐

(e) Surgical intervention is effective and evidence-based ☐ ☐

9.9 Vulvovaginal candidiasis

(a) Is usually associated with itching and vaginal discharge ☐ ☐

(b) Is rarely caused by antibiotic therapy ☐ ☐

(c) Can be a presenting symptom of diabetes mellitus ☐ ☐

(d) Is not transmitted to the male sexual partner ☐ ☐

(e) Is treated with an intravaginal imidazole as the drug of first choice ☐ ☐

9.10 Infertility T F

(a) 5–10% of normal fertile couples take more than a year to conceive ☐ ☐

(b) Sperm dysfunction, ovulation disorder and fallopian tube damage are the top three causes ☐ ☐

(c) No definite cause is found in over 50% of couples ☐ ☐

(d) Metformin can be used for treating polycystic ovary syndrome ☐ ☐

(e) Clomiphene can only be prescribed by a hospital specialist ☐ ☐

9.11 Unintended pregnancy in young women

(a) Early child bearing has a negative association with health outcomes ☐ ☐

(b) Adolescent females want more advice on negotiation skills in sexual relationships ☐ ☐

(c) Initiation of sexual intercourse can be prevented by patient education in primary care ☐ ☐

(d) There is good evidence from randomised controlled trials that improved use of birth control can be achieved by education ☐ ☐

(e) Incidence is lower in the Netherlands than in the UK ☐ ☐

9.12 Uterovaginal prolapse

(a) Does not cause problems with sexual activity ☐ ☐

(b) Is known to decrease in incidence after hysterectomy ☐ ☐

(c) Can cause ulceration of the cervix ☐ ☐

(d) May be aggravated by pelvic floor exercises ☐ ☐

(e) Is treated by vaginal hysterectomy as the treatment of choice ☐ ☐

9.13 Breast cancer

(a) BRAC1 and BRAC2 genes are responsible for over 50% of cases ☐ ☐

	T	F

(b) Prophylactic treatment with tamoxifen can be used for high-risk cases ☐ ☐

(c) With axillary dissection, a sentinel node can be found in more than 90% of patients ☐ ☐

(d) Metastases can be treated with anti-oestrogens in premenopausal but not postmenopausal patients ☐ ☐

(e) Chemotherapy has no role in the modern treatment of disseminated disease ☐ ☐

9.14 Mother-to-child transmission of HIV

(a) Transmission rates are as high as one in three ☐ ☐

(b) Antiretroviral treatment for the mother does not reduce the risk to the child ☐ ☐

(c) Breast feeding should be encouraged ☐ ☐

(d) Elective Caesarean section can reduce the risk of transmission by half ☐ ☐

(e) If the mother dies her baby is more likely to die in infancy ☐ ☐

9.15 Hormone replacement therapy (HRT)

a) Should be offered to women for prevention of cardiovascular disease ☐ ☐

b) Is associated with a significantly increased risk of breast cancer after two years of use ☐ ☐

c) Can prevent osteoporosis caused by steroid therapy ☐ ☐

d) Results in greatest increase in risk of pulmonary embolism in the first year of use ☐ ☐

e) Decreases the risk of endometrial cancer in the long term ☐ ☐

9.16 Pre-term labour

(a) There is an association with lethal foetal malformations ☐ ☐

T F

(b) Prostaglandin–synthetase inhibitors are contraindicated ☐ ☐

(c) Antepartum haemorrhage may precipitate the event ☐ ☐

(d) Membrane rupture contraindicates use of glucocorticoid drugs in the mother ☐ ☐

(e) Routine episiotomy is recommended ☐ ☐

9.17 Progestogen-containing contraceptives

(a) The progestogen-releasing IUD may cause increased vaginal blood loss ☐ ☐

(b) The progesterone-only pill is unsuitable for lactating mothers ☐ ☐

(c) Patients on long-term hepatic enzyme–inducing drugs may need higher doses of the progesterone-only pill ☐ ☐

(d) Injectable progestogens may increase HDL cholesterol ☐ ☐

(e) The levonorgestrel-releasing implant lasts for five years ☐ ☐

9.18 Multiple pregnancy

(a) The incidence of twins is approximately one in ninety pregnancies ☐ ☐

(b) Pregnancy-induced hypertension is more common, but generally mild ☐ ☐

(c) Hydramnios is a complication in about 5% ☐ ☐

(d) The risks of cerebral palsy in the neonate are higher ☐ ☐

(e) Hospital admission for bed rest for the mother produces significantly better outcomes for the neonate ☐ ☐

9.19 Managing gestational diabetes

(a) Insulin does not cross the placenta but glucose and other metabolites do ☐ ☐

T   F

(b) Oral hypoglycaemic agents may be used if hyperglycaemia is not severe ☐ ☐

(c) 40% of women with gestational diabetes will develop Type 2 diabetes within twenty years ☐ ☐

(d) Treatment can usually be discontinued postpartum, as the condition generally resolves ☐ ☐

(e) There is little correlation between HbA1c in early pregnancy and congenital abnormalities ☐ ☐

Section 10

Growth and development

10.1 Infantile colic

		T	F
(a)	Starts in the first few weeks of life and ends by four to five months	☐	☐
(b)	Causes one in six families to consult a health professional	☐	☐
(c)	Is less common in breast-fed babies	☐	☐
(d)	Is associated with poor parenting skills	☐	☐
(e)	Antimuscarinic drugs have few adverse effects	☐	☐

10.2 Enuresis

(a)	Daytime urinary symptoms suggest underlying bladder dysfunction	☐	☐
(b)	Alarms are not an effective treatment	☐	☐
(c)	Desmospressin has lasting benefit after treatment is stopped	☐	☐
(d)	Imipramine is safe and rarely causes adverse effects in children	☐	☐
(e)	Can be precipitated by stress	☐	☐

10.3 Characteristic features of gonadal dysgenesis (Turner's syndrome) include

(a)	XO Sex chromosome pattern	☐	☐
(b)	Decreased urinary gonadotrophins (FSH) after puberty	☐	☐
(c)	Abnormal female genitalia	☐	☐
(d)	Webbing of the neck	☐	☐
(e)	Short fourth metacarpal	☐	☐

10.4 The following apply to child care legislation in the United Kingdom

T F

(a) An Emergency Protection Order lasts for twenty-eight days ☐ ☐

(b) Parental consent is required before Care or Supervision Orders can be applied ☐ ☐

(c) Police protection provisions require a warrant ☐ ☐

(d) Children are counted as being in need of local authority services if they are permanently disabled by congenital deformity or mental disorder, unless the disability is restricted to deafness. ☐ ☐

(e) The Children's Act (1989) requires the child's consent to examination if he is of sufficient understanding to make an informed decision ☐ ☐

10.5 In the management of febrile convulsions

(a) The child should be kept in the supine position to facilitate observation ☐ ☐

(b) Rectal diazepam produces an effective blood concentration of anticonvulsant within ten minutes ☐ ☐

(c) Children with a first febrile convulsion may be managed at home if the parents appear educated ☐ ☐

(d) It is important to exclude meningitis by lumbar puncture if the child is less than eighteen months old ☐ ☐

(e) Phenobarbitone should be used in prevention in most cases ☐ ☐

10.6 Low birth weight babies

(a) Are defined as those weighing less than 2 kg at birth ☐ ☐

(b) Generally look wasted if born small-for-dates at term ☐ ☐

(c) Commonly suffer from necrotizing enterocolitis after the third week of life ☐ ☐

(d) Are more commonly born to mothers who have suffered toxoplasmosis whilst pregnant ☐ ☐

	T	F
(e) Characteristically have lanugo body hair if preterm	☐	☐

10.7 Breathholding attacks

	T	F
(a) May include clonic movements lasting a few seconds	☐	☐
(b) Usually begin at nine to eighteen months	☐	☐
(c) Are characterised by cyanotic spells which are commonly precipitated by frustration and rage	☐	☐
(d) Are successfully prevented by the use of anticonvulsants and sedatives	☐	☐
(e) Terminate with the child taking a deep breath and regaining consciousness over the next five minutes	☐	☐

10.8 By the eighth month of life an infant would be expected to

	T	F
(a) Give a brick to his parent	☐	☐
(b) Feed himself with a biscuit	☐	☐
(c) Walk holding onto furniture	☐	☐
(d) Turn his head to a sound above the level of the ear	☐	☐
(e) Say one word with meaning	☐	☐

10.9 Breast milk is better than modified cow's milk formula for infant feeding because

	T	F
(a) It is richer in calories	☐	☐
(b) Less likely to result in jaundice	☐	☐
(c) It contains more protein	☐	☐
(d) The composition of the milk is consistent throughout feeding	☐	☐
(e) It is less likely to cause hypocalcaemic tetany	☐	☐

10.10 Gastroenteritis in infants living in the United Kingdom   T   F

(a) Is more common in breast-fed babies   ☐ ☐

(b) Is commonly caused by Campylobacter   ☐ ☐

(c) Is typically associated with a preceding history of recurrent colic   ☐ ☐

(d) May be treated with dicyclomine   ☐ ☐

(e) Requires specialist review if bowel movements become bloody   ☐ ☐

10.11 The Apgar score designed to assess the degree of respiratory depression in a neonate requires assessment of

(a) Heart rate   ☐ ☐

(b) Cough reflex   ☐ ☐

(c) Muscle tone   ☐ ☐

(d) Respiratory effort   ☐ ☐

(e) Colour   ☐ ☐

10.12 Childhood injuries

(a) Are much commoner in social classes 1 and 2 than in social classes 4 and 5   ☐ ☐

(b) Needing admission are most commonly due to accidental overdose   ☐ ☐

(c) In car passengers are reduced by use of standard seat belts   ☐ ☐

(d) Are strongly associated with child neglect   ☐ ☐

(e) May be prevented by health visitor intervention   ☐ ☐

10.13 Developmental delay

(a) Affects at least 5% of the UK under fives   ☐ ☐

(b) Is generally more severe if due to environmental causes   ☐ ☐

	T	F

(c)   Is associated with malnutrition ☐ ☐

(d)   Can be caused by parental alcohol abuse ☐ ☐

(e)   Can be prevented for some conditions by routine screening methods ☐ ☐

10.14 Acute abdominal pain in children

(a)   Is a known consequence of inflamed lymph nodes in the region of the terminal ileum ☐ ☐

(b)   Requiring surgical intervention is most commonly due to intussusception ☐ ☐

(c)   Is more likely to have a medical than surgical cause if vomiting precedes the pain ☐ ☐

(d)   Is a common feature of childhood migraine ☐ ☐

(e)   The most valuable imaging technique is ultrasound scanning ☐ ☐

10.15 Risk factors for hearing loss include

(a)   Infants requiring intensive care ☐ ☐

(b)   Meningitis ☐ ☐

(c)   Congenital toxoplasmosis ☐ ☐

(d)   Tetracycline treatment ☐ ☐

(e)   Congenital cytomegalovirus infection ☐ ☐

10.16 Squint in children

(a)   May be the only outward sign of serious eye disease ☐ ☐

(b)   May be a normal variation in children up to the age of three years ☐ ☐

(c)   Is always abnormal if uniocular ☐ ☐

(d)   May cause amblyopia ☐ ☐

	T	F
(e) Is a common complication of premature birth	☐	☐

10.17 In assessing a child's language development

	T	F
(a) Girls talk earlier and have a larger vocabulary than boys up to the age of three	☐	☐
(b) The number and positioning of siblings is not related to rate of language acquisition	☐	☐
(c) Bilingual children are generally slightly delayed in the development of both languages compared to monolingual peers	☐	☐
(d) A child not interested in stories at age three years is delayed	☐	☐
(e) Maternal depression is associated with delayed language acquisition	☐	☐

10.18 Deafness after birth may follow

(a) Otitis media in neonate	☐	☐
(b) Rubella in pregnancy	☐	☐
(c) Neonatal hyperbilirubinaemia	☐	☐
(d) Severe perinatal anoxia	☐	☐
(e) Drug treatment in the neonatal period (for example with streptomycin, kanamycin or gentamicin)	☐	☐

10.19 Neonatal screening in the United Kingdom is routine in all children whose parents consent for the following conditions

(a) Sickle cell trait	☐	☐
(b) Phenylketonuria	☐	☐
(c) Galactosaemia	☐	☐
(d) Strabismus	☐	☐
(e) Urinary tract infection	☐	☐

10.20 The following are facts about skull growth in childhood   T   F

(a)   The anterior fontanelle should never be patent at one year of age   ☐   ☐

(b)   Premature craniostenosis may occur as an isolated congenital deformity   ☐   ☐

(c)   Infants suspected of having craniostenosis do not need referral before two years before definite treatment   ☐   ☐

(d)   Macrocephaly is seldom associated with mental handicap   ☐   ☐

(e)   Turner's syndrome is a rare cause of oxycephaly   ☐   ☐

Section 11

The mind

11.1 People who self-harm

                                                                     T   F

(a) Should always be assessed for suicidal risk   ☐ ☐

(b) A multidisciplinary team approach to assessment and management is optimal   ☐ ☐

(c) It is usually not necessary to involve a psychiatrist   ☐ ☐

(d) Self-harm is ten to twenty times more frequent than suicide   ☐ ☐

(e) Previous episodes do not increase the risk of suicide   ☐ ☐

11.2 Bulimia nervosa

(a) Cognitive behavioural therapy is likely to be beneficial   ☐ ☐

(b) Antidepressants (eg. SSRIs) are of minimal benefit   ☐ ☐

(c) Binge eating and purgative behaviour are usually easy to identify   ☐ ☐

(d) Weight can be normal   ☐ ☐

(e) Is equally common in men and women   ☐ ☐

11.3 Non-cardiac chest pain of psychological causation

(a) Half of the patients referred from general practice to a cardiac clinic with chest pain and palpitations do not have cardiac disease   ☐ ☐

(b) Despite the absence of cardiac disease, over two thirds have long term symptoms   ☐ ☐

(c) Panic attacks are commonly associated   ☐ ☐

(d) Depression is uncommon   ☐ ☐

T F

(e) As few as three questions can differentiate most patients with chest pain who have coronary heart disease from those who do not ☐ ☐

11.4 Anxiety

(a) Generalised anxiety disorder, panic disorder, and phobic anxiety have a prevalence of 5% in the general adult population ☐ ☐

(b) Is commonly associated with sense of difficulty breathing ☐ ☐

(c) Feeling dizzy, unsteady, faint, or light headed is uncommon ☐ ☐

(d) The hospital anxiety and depression scale is better at detecting depression than anxiety ☐ ☐

(e) Can be caused by SSRIs ☐ ☐

11.5 Depression

(a) Major depressive disorder affects one in twenty people during their lifetime ☐ ☐

(b) Is rarely associated with physical illness ☐ ☐

(c) Can be a presenting feature of alcoholism ☐ ☐

(d) Is more common in men than in women ☐ ☐

(e) Is associated with greater mortality after myocardial infarction ☐ ☐

11.6 Age-related memory loss

(a) 40% of people aged sixty-five or more have memory impairment ☐ ☐

(b) The risk remains constant with increasing age ☐ ☐

(c) Cerebrovascular disease and Alzheimer's disease do not occur together ☐ ☐

(d) Cognitive impairment can be detected with a simple screening questionnaire ☐ ☐

T   F

(e) The risk of memory loss is higher in those who have been intellectually active ☐ ☐

11.7 Bipolar mood disorder

(a) Suicide is not a significant concern ☐ ☐

(b) The life time prevalence is more than 1% ☐ ☐

(c) Lithium is no longer the first choice for prophylactic treatment ☐ ☐

(d) Sodium valproate is used in routine treatment ☐ ☐

(e) Regular screening for hyperthyroidism is needed in patients taking lithium ☐ ☐

11.8 Tardive dyskinesia

(a) Is characterised by lipsmacking and periorbital tics ☐ ☐

(b) Is a recognised complication of long-term use of chlorpromazine, but not of trifluoperazine ☐ ☐

(c) Would be expected to resolve completely if the dose of antipsychotic drugs was reduced ☐ ☐

(d) May be ameliorated by anticholinergic preparations in adequate dose ☐ ☐

(e) Is a variant of the movement disorder hemiballismus ☐ ☐

11.9 Children with autism

(a) Characteristically show impairments in reciprocal social interaction ☐ ☐

(b) Often show repetitive, stereotyped behaviour patterns ☐ ☐

(c) Are more likely to have mothers who are cold and indifferent to their infants ☐ ☐

(d) Show an association with extremes of head size ☐ ☐

(e) Are unlikely to be genetically predisposed to the condition ☐ ☐

11.10 When a patient is admitted compulsorily to a hospital in England under the Mental Health Act (1983) the following apply   T   F

(a) Recommendation for admission under Section 3 requires two doctors approved under section 12

(b) Compulsory treatment may be given up to tw days after admission under Section 2

(c) Treatment for any physical illness falls outside the remit of the Mental Health Act

(d) Section 4 allows for emergency treatment of mental conditions for up to seventy-two hours from admission

(e) Patient or relatives may apply to a Mental Health Review Tribunal but only within the first fourteen days of detention

11.11 Risk factors for schizophrenia include

(a) High socio-economic status

(b) Small size at birth for gestational age

(c) A positive family history

(d) Female gender

(e) Cannabis use in adolescence

11.12 Cannabis

(a) The presence of signs of papillary constriction and hypothermia in users should be regarded as a medical emergency

(b) It may be prescribed by doctors for its analgesic effects on a named patient basis

(c) Up to 10% of adolescents have used cannabis by the age of twenty

(d) Depression and anxiety in teenagers predict later cannabis use

(e) Regular use substantially increases the risk of major depression

11.13 Factors associated with increased risk of suicide include

                                                                       T   F

(a) Delusions of immortality

(b) Female gender

(c) Sexual disinhibition

(d) Slowing of thoughts

(e) A recent visit to a psychiatrist

11.14 Patients who abuse alcohol

(a) Have a 10% mortality risk if delirium tremens is untreated

(b) In general, will develop diabetes mellitus before retirement age

(c) Have a higher than average risk of oral cancers

(d) Can be given chlormethiazole to prevent a withdrawal syndrome

(e) Are protected against coronary artery disease

11.15 Patients with anorexia nervosa

(a) May present with primary amenorrhoea

(b) Benefit from cognitive behaviour therapy

(c) Are reluctant to prepare food for others

(d) Have a mortality in the order of 1–2%

(e) May have hyperkalaemia, if self-induced vomiting is frequent

11.16 Drug addiction and dependence

(a) Is commoner for legal than illegal substances

(b) Is commoner in men than women

(c) Is diagnosed in part by evidence of altered behaviour to accommodate the need to prioritise obtaining the drug

T   F

(d) For heroin and cocaine, requires NHS staff to notify local police of user details ☐ ☐

(e) May present as an acute psychotic state ☐ ☐

11.17 Women with Down's syndrome are at greater risk of

(a) Congenital heart problems ☐ ☐

(b) Subfertility ☐ ☐

(c) Visual impairment ☐ ☐

(d) Poorly controlled epilepsy ☐ ☐

(e) Underuse of well woman services ☐ ☐

11.18 Medically unexplained symptoms

(a) Are often attributed by patients to a causal event ☐ ☐

(b) Are associated with lower socioeconomic status ☐ ☐

(c) Patients have a lower incidence of anger compared to patients who are adjusting to a known diagnosis ☐ ☐

(d) Are associated with malignant disease ☐ ☐

(e) Increased incidence in depression ☐ ☐

11.19 Attention deficit hyperactivity disorder

(a) Incidence is around 3% ☐ ☐

(b) Only 20% of these children will have seen their GP in the last year ☐ ☐

(c) Questionnaires are more specific in aiding diagnosis than consultation ☐ ☐

(d) Diet contributes to the condition in approximately 20% of cases ☐ ☐

(e) The condition is probably underdiagnosed ☐ ☐

Section 12

Emergency medicine

12.1 Chemical weapons   T   F

   (a) Were developed after World War II   ☐ ☐

   (b) Poisoning with many chemical agents, especially nerve agents, cannot be treated even when diagnosed early   ☐ ☐

   (c) Decontamination is the first priority   ☐ ☐

   (d) Nerve agents act by inhibiting acetylcholinesterase   ☐ ☐

   (e) Severe pulmonary oedema can occur several hours after contact with phosgene   ☐ ☐

12.2 Emergency medicine

   (a) Overcrowding in Accident and Emergency departments is the biggest impediment to the delivery of care   ☐ ☐

   (b) Amiodarone is the antiarrhythmic drug of choice for cardiac arrest due to shock refractory ventricular fibrillation or ventricular tachycardia   ☐ ☐

   (c) Death is common after an overdose of atypical antipsychotic agents   ☐ ☐

   (d) Neck injury in a patient who is intoxicated is an indication for a cervical X-ray   ☐ ☐

   (e) A Glasgow coma score of less than fifteen at two hours after a head injury indicates a high risk for surgical intervention   ☐ ☐

12.3 Road traffic accidents

   (a) Seat belts offer less protection than air bags   ☐ ☐

   (b) Most school age children wear seat belts   ☐ ☐

T   F

(c) Acute sleepiness significantly increases the risk of a RTA in which the car occupant is injured or killed ☐ ☐

(d) Morbidity in young children is greater in lower socio-economic groups ☐ ☐

(e) Intravenous infusion may cause more harm than good ☐ ☐

12.4 Dengue fever

(a) Is the most common arboviral disease ☐ ☐

(b) The prevalence is decreasing ☐ ☐

(c) Is characterised by haemorrhagic fever ☐ ☐

(d) The vector, Aedes Aegypti, occurs in African countries bordering on the Mediterranean Sea ☐ ☐

(e) Can be prevented with a specific vaccine ☐ ☐

12.5 Travel medicine

(a) Refugees and migrants have a higher incidence of tuberculosis ☐ ☐

(b) Malaria is the single most important serious disease hazard facing travellers ☐ ☐

(c) Hepatitis A and B vaccines are recommended for travel to Australia and New Zealand ☐ ☐

(d) Deep vein thrombosis is a risk on short distance flights ☐ ☐

(e) Meningococcal meningitis is a risk on pilgrimages in the Middle East ☐ ☐

12.6 Acute pancreatitis

(a) Gallstones and alcohol are common causes ☐ ☐

(b) Can be iatrogenic ☐ ☐

(c) Does not cause retroperitoneal bleeding ☐ ☐

	T	F

(d) Serum amylase over three times normal is diagnostic ☐ ☐

(e) Mortality has decreased over the last twenty years ☐ ☐

12.7 Taking a drug overdose

(a) Is less likely to be associated with a serious suicide attempt than physical methods such as attempted hanging ☐ ☐

(b) May be accidental ☐ ☐

(c) Will need a prolonged period of observation for possible side-effects ☐ ☐

(d) Is less likely to be of prescribed than over-the-counter or illegal drugs ☐ ☐

(e) May be associated with being a victim of domestic violence ☐ ☐

12.8 In shock

(a) A drop in systolic blood pressure below 90 indicates a loss 15% in blood volume ☐ ☐

(b) In anaphylactic shock adrenaline is best given subcutaneously ☐ ☐

(c) Stabilising the neck in a person after a head on collision is secondary importance to assessing the pulse ☐ ☐

(d) Three times the volume of crystalline fluid is needed for each volume of blood lost ☐ ☐

(e) A sling under a fractured pelvis can help reduce blood loss ☐ ☐

12.9 After an episode of syncope

(a) 15% of drivers immediately stop driving ☐ ☐

(b) Counselling about driving after such an event is effective in reducing the number of patients who continue to drive ☐ ☐

(c) 9% of drivers who are injured in an accident caused by their syncopal episode stop driving in the short term. ☐ ☐

T   F

(d) After one episode of syncope the DLVA recommends to stop driving until diagnosis and/or treatment initiated ☐ ☐

(e) A diagnosis may not be made in up to 40% of episodes of syncope ☐ ☐

12.10 Thiazide diuretics may interact adversely with the following drugs

(a) Amiodarone

☐ ☐

(b) Spironolactone

☐ ☐

(c) Chlorpropamide

☐ ☐

(d) Indomethacin

☐ ☐

(e) Macrolide antibiotics

☐ ☐

12.11 The following are recognised causes of drug-induced asthma

(a) Ibuprofen

(b) Calcium channel-blockers ☐ ☐

(c) Paracetamol ☐ ☐

(d) Angiotensin converting enzyme inhibitors ☐ ☐

(e) Propellants used in salbutamol metered-dose inhalers ☐ ☐

☐ ☐

12.12 The calcium channel blocker nifedipine

(a) Has a useful therapeutic anti-arrhythmic effect

(b) Should not be used with beta-blockers ☐ ☐

(c) Is particularly valuable in the first month after myocardial infarction ☐ ☐

(d) May cause ischaemic cardiac pain within half-an-hour of starting the drug ☐ ☐

☐ ☐

	T	F

(e) May be used to manage Raynaud's phenomenon ☐ ☐

12.13 Spontaneous pneumothorax

(a) Usually follows an acute respiratory infection ☐ ☐

(b) More often affects the left lung than the right ☐ ☐

(c) Occurs more often in males ☐ ☐

(d) May be triggered by high altitude flying ☐ ☐

(e) Presents with sharp pain on inspiration with or without dyspnoea ☐ ☐

12.14 Anaphylaxis

(a) A working definition should include both respiratory difficulty and hypotension. ☐ ☐

(b) Drugs are the second most common cause of anaphylaxis ☐ ☐

(c) Reactions to latex occur over about thirty minutes ☐ ☐

(d) Mast cell tryptase can be used as an immediate investigation ☐ ☐

(e) Reporting of MI after using adrenaline for treatment probably reflects a bias in reporting ☐ ☐

12.15 Pulmonary embolus

(a) Pulmonary angiography is the gold standard investigation ☐ ☐

(b) Ventilation perfusion scans are diagnostic in only 30% cases ☐ ☐

(c) Warfarin is the first treatment step ☐ ☐

(d) A normal non-invasive investigation of leg veins is significant in excluding the likelihood of pulmonary embolus ☐ ☐

(e) D-dimer is a fragment of the fibrinolytic system ☐ ☐

12.16 Paediatric burns   T   F

(a) 18% of paediatric burns are as a result of using bowls of water to heat bottles for feeding babies

☐ ☐

(b) Heating milk for bottle feeding increases rate of gastric emptying

☐ ☐

(c) Most paediatric units in the UK do not routinely heat milk for bottle feeding

☐ ☐

(d) Microwaves pose less of a risk of burning than conventional ovens

☐ ☐

(e) Burns from heating of milk in bowls of water is well publicised

☐ ☐

12.17 Drowning

(a) Over half of deaths worldwide are in the under fourteen years

☐ ☐

(b) Is the most common cause of childhood death

☐ ☐

(c) In recent years there has been an increase in drowning in freshwater sites such as lakes and rivers

☐ ☐

(d) Ability to swim reduces death by drowning

☐ ☐

(e) Fencing around swimming pools is the only effective intervention to reduce drowning

☐ ☐

Part 2
Extended matching questions

Introduction

The main part of this book has been devoted to multiple 'true/false' questions, a familiar format for many tutors and students. However, these questions often place undue emphasis on recall, and when a student answers a 'false' question correctly, it can only be concluded that the student knew the statement was false – nothing can be deduced about what the student does know (Schuwirth and van der Vleuten, 2003).

Many medical assessments now use the type of question called extended matching questions (EMQs). These include the postgraduate knowledge paper for GP vocational training summative assessment, and the Professional and Linguistics Assessment Board (PLAB) test (MacDonald, 2001) (which is used to assess non-UK medical graduates for work in the UK). Other postgraduate medical examinations are using the EMQ format, and there are similar trends in undergraduate examinations, and internationally.

EMQs differ from true/false MCQs, insofar that the student must integrate several pieces of information, thus testing higher order cognitive skills such as application of knowledge, interpretation of data, and problem-solving ability. Although each question may take longer to answer than standard MCQs, a two-hour exam paper can achieve acceptable coverage and reliability.

EMQs provide the student with a list of options, a stem question, or some clinical vignettes, which emphasise the clinical relevance of the information. Extended matching sets usually include the following four elements:

~ a theme
~ an option list
~ a lead-in statement
~ a number of item stems.

The themes may be quite varied, with a number of options forming the list of potential answers. Item stems are often written as the clinical vignette, with the lead-in statement providing direction to the student. By way of example, labels have been attached to the four elements of the EMQ on blood pressure measurement, the first EMQ in the section.

When answering an extended matching question, remember that one of its options may be correct for more than one of its vignettes, and some options may be 'distractors', not applying to any of the vignettes — this is to reduce the chances of gaining marks by guessing. When answering EMQs, first try to identify the clinical problem (if not already given), and then think of your own list of possible diagnoses that could cause the problem, or possible solutions to the problem given. Finally, look at the list of options to see whether there is an equivalent option to your own intuitive choice of answer.

The examples in this section aim to give the student an idea of the range of EMQs that may be encountered in examinations today. It is not intended that they cover all clinical areas that could be tested, or show all the possible formats. They are set at varying levels of difficulty. The first EMQ, on blood pressure measurement, is aimed at undergraduate level. The remaining questions are aimed somewhere between undergraduate and postgraduate level.

References

MacDonald R (2001) The PLAB test: separating the facts from the fiction. *Br Med J* **322**: S2–7292

Schuwirth LWT, van der Vleuten CPM (2003) ABC of learning and teaching in medicine: Written assessment. *Br Med J* **326**: 643–5

EMQs: questions

EMQ 1: Measurement of blood pressure (theme)

Read the passage below on blood pressure measurement and fill in the gaps with the most appropriate word from the list below. Words may be used more than once, or not at all.

Considerable variability occurs in blood pressure from moment to moment and it may (1)_____ with bladder distension or pain. It is usually at its (2)_____ during sleep. (3)_____ may raise blood pressure by as much as 30mm Hg and is usually reduced or abolished with (4)_____ and familiarity by the doctor with the technique and circumstances of blood pressure measurement.

Posture affects blood pressure, with a general tendency for it to (5)_____ from the lying to the sitting or standing position. The arm should also be supported at (6)_____ level. Dependency of the arm below this level leads to a/an (7)_____ of systolic and diastolic pressures and raising the arm above this level leads to (8)_____. If the measuring cuff is too small this leads to a/an (9)_____ of blood pressure; if too large then a/an (10)_____ of blood pressure will result. (11)_____ is more common than (12)_____.

(13)_____ hypertension is a condition in which a normotensive subject becomes hypertensive during blood pressure measurement, but pressures then settle to normal outside the medical environment. The true blood pressure values are best demonstrated by (14)_____.

ambulatory blood pressure measurement	nurses
anxiety	overcuffing
coffee	overestimation
decrease	pseudohypertension
desk	reassurance
gestational	shoulder smoking
heart	undercuffing
highest	underestimation
hospital monitoring	white coat
increase	white collar
lowest	

EMQ 2: Hypertension

In the management of hypertension, match the following target levels of blood pressure with the most appropriate description of the evidence or guidelines.

1   140/90 mmHg
2   144/82 mmHg
3   135/75 mmHg
4   134/84 mmHg
5   150/90 mmHg

A   The UK Prospective Diabetes Study (UKPDS) found that in this intensive blood pressure treatment group, diabetics had a 34% reduction in macrovascular complications and a 37% reduction in microvascular complications

B   NICE guidelines target BP for the treatment of hypertension in type 2 diabetics with microalbuminuria

C   Represents the audit standard for treatment of hypertension in an adult without other risk factors

D   British Hypertension Society in patients with NIDDM, anti-hypertensive treatment should be started when blood pressure exceeds this level

E   If found in an adult without other risk factors, recommendations are to repeat the reading in five years as this level would be considered acceptable

EMQ 3: Visual disturbance

A   Ophthalmic migraine
B   Retinal detachment
C   Dysthyroid eye disease
D   Acute angle closure glaucoma
E   Retinal artery occlusion
F   Anterior uveitis (iridocyclitis)
G   Horner's syndrome
H   Age-related macular degeneration
I   Pituitary tumour
J   Conjunctivitis
K   Cataract
L   Retrobulbar neuritis

For each description of visual disturbance below, select the most likely diagnosis.

1   Vision worsens in bright light; diminished red reflex on ophthalmoscopy

2   Gradual central field loss, pigmentary changes at the macula

3   Bitemporal field defect, afferent papillary defect

4   Blurred vision, painful red eye improved by going to sleep

5   Central field loss, red desaturation; painful eye, worse on movement

6   Floaters and flashing lights; variable acuity and field loss

7   Photophobia, eye pain worsened by reading; red eye

8   'Curtain' descending over the vision, cherry-red appearance of the macula

EMQ 4: Musculoskeletal disorders

A   Pes planus and Morton's metatarsalgia
B   Plantar fasciitis
C   Fracture of the second metatarsal
D   Fracture of the calcaneum
E   Osteochondritis of the navicular (Kohler's disease)
F   Apophysitis of the calcaneum (Sever's disease)
G   Rheumatoid arthritis
H   Osteoarthritis
I   Gout

Thinking about the diagnosis of foot pain, match the above diagnoses to the most likely clinical scenario

1   A thirty-year-old florist with painful swollen metatarsal joints, clawing of the toes, and effusions

2   A five-year-old child limping with a painful foot

3   A middle-aged porter with pain along the inner border of the heel, worse on putting his foot to the ground first thing in the morning

4   A retired man with a gradually worsening painful stiff metatarsal joint of the first toe

5   A twenty-year-old secretary with pain in the forefoot, worse on weight-bearing, after returning from a sponsored walk

6   A young man who has jumped off a wall, who also complains of back pain

7   A middle-aged woman who needs wider-fitting shoes has a painful spot in her forefoot, and numbness of the adjacent parts of two of the toes

8   A middle-aged businessman returning after a long haul flight with an acutely painful metatarsal joint of the first toe

9   A teenager with a painful heel now prevented from sprinting

EMQ 5: Herbal remedies

Match the most appropriate pharmacological effect to each herbal remedy below. Each option may be used only once.

1   St John's wort
2   Echinacea
3   Gingko biloba
4   Saw palmetto
5   Kava kava
6   Liquorice
7   Evening primrose oil

A   Can cause antagonism of diuretic effect of Spironolactone

B   Can cause altered bleeding time with warfarin

C   Has been shown to have a beneficial effect in the treatment of the common cold

D   Can cause lowered seizure threshold in patients on anticonvulsants

E   Can cause additive sedative effects with benzodiazepines

F   Has been shown to have a beneficial effect in the treatment of benign prostatic hyperplasia

G   Has been shown to have a beneficial effect in the treatment of depression

EMQ 6: Bowel disorders

Match each of the following bowel conditions with the three most likely symptoms or clinical features.

1   Inflammatory bowel disease
2   Colonic cancer
3   Irritable bowel disorder

A   Age greater than fifty

B   Abdominal fullness, bloating, or swelling

C   Mouth ulcers and anal tags

D   Fever and malaise

E   Abdominal pain relieved by defecation

F   Iron deficiency anaemia with normal stools

G   Hard or lumpy stools

H   Rectal bleeding starting after giving up smoking

I   Large flat adenomas

EMQ 7: Oral contraception

Read the passage below and fill in the gaps with the most appropriate word from the list below. Words may be used more than once, or not at all.

Women today are faced with many choices concerning oral contraception. Absolute contraindications to the combined pill include (1)_____ and (2)_____. Relative contraindications include (3)_____, and a family history of (4)_____. Progestogens such as desogestrel are less (5)_____ than the older progestogens, and do not have the adverse effect on blood lipids seen with levonogestrel. They do, however, carry an increased risk of (6)_____. The more (7)_____ pills may increase the risk of coronary heart disease three-fold. Women on the combined pill should be warned that there is a possible increased risk of cancer of the (8)_____ and (9)_____, although there is a reduction in risk of cancer of the (10)_____and the (11)_____. Patients with persistent breakthrough bleeding can be tried on a/an (12)_____ pill, or by reducing the pill-free interval using the (13)_____ method. Phased preparations are more likely to cause (14)_____ symptoms towards the end of the pack. Other side-effects of combined pills with a relative oestrogen excess include (15)_____ and (16)_____. Side-effects of combined pills with a relative progestogen excess include (17)_____ and (18)_____.

androgenic	ovary
arterial thrombo-embolism	phlebitis
breast	premenstrual tension
cervix	psychogenic
chronic liver disease	purulent vaginal discharge
cost-effective	renal stones
deep vein thrombosis	sickle cell trait
endometrium	stomach
hirsutism	thyroid gland
large bowel	tricycle
loss of libido	triphasic
lung	triangle
nausea	vaginal discharge without infection
obesity	vulva
oestrogenic	

EMQ 8: Musculoskeletal disorders

A   ESR greater than 50 mm/hr
B   Rheumatoid factor positive
C   Bone density average T score of minus 2.9 or below
D   Peri-articular osteopenia
E   C reactive protein of 20
F   Degenerative changes and osteophytes on cervical spine X-ray
G   Chronic back pain

For each description of a clinical case below, select the most likely diagnosis or positive investigative finding from the list of options above. An option may be used once, more than once, or not at all. Cases may be matched with up to two options per case.

1   A young man with inflamed small joints of the hands and wrists, three months after travelling to India, where he had an acute diarrhoea episode

2   A lady of fifty-nine years who has gradually developed shoulder upper arm and neck pain, and is feeling tired

3   Associated with polymyalgia rheumatica

4   Present in at least 15% of the population

5   A lady who has two days previously suffered a rear shunt road traffic accident, and has acute neck pain

6   Best treated with oral bisphosphonates

7   Associated with smoking

8   Associated with long standing rheumatoid arthritis

EMQ 9: Musculoskeletal disorders

A   Plantar fasciitis
B   Low back pain
C   Carpal tunnel syndrome
D   Anterior knee pain
E   Hallux valgus
F   Pronated ankle
G   Bicipital tendonitis
H   Achilles tendonitis

For each statement below, select the appropriate diagnosis(es) from the list of options above. An option may be used once, more than once, or not at all. Up to three options may be used per case.

1   Conditions for which a heel raise could be helpful

2   Can be treated with manipulation

3   Effective treatments include arch supports

4   Depo-medrone injection can aid recovery

5   Found in ankylosing spondylitis

6   Associated with recreational running

EMQ 10: Ear, nose and throat symptoms

A   Chronic otitis externa
B   Acute otitis media
C   Ear wax
D   Chronic suppurative otitis media
E   Perforated tympanic membrane
F   Vertigo

For each statement below, select the appropriate diagnosis(es) from the list of options above. An option may be used once, more than once, or not at all. Up to three options may be used per case.

1   Incidence is about 1%

2   Incidence rises at the end of the summer

3   Has been shown to cause itchiness in ear

4   More likely to be present if there is a smoker in the household

5   Increased incidence in females

6   Can be treated with surgery

7   Hearing loss is usually the presenting symptom

8   Is a complication of ear syringing

EMQ 11: Infections in primary care

A   In the majority of patients symptoms are relieved by three days antibiotics

B   A ten-day course of antibiotics has been shown to reduce recurrence

C   The majority of patients do not consult their GP for this condition

D   Microscopy and culture can improve outcome

E   Significant antibiotic resistance occurs in the UK

F   Culture demonstrates that over 50% of the population can be carriers of organism implicated in infection

G   Non-antibiotic treatments have been shown to increase incidence of adverse effects

H   Risk of anaphylaxis from antibiotics is greater than risk of complications of infection

I   Commonest reason for consulting a GP

J   20% of patients re-consult for continuing symptoms

For each statement above, select the appropriate diagnosis(es) from the list of options below. An option may be used once, more than once, or not at all. Up to four options may be used per case.

1   Acute otitis media
2   Uncomplicated urinary tract infection
3   Complicated urinary tract infection
4   Sore throat
5   Pustular tonsillitis
6   Impetigo
7   Lower respiratory tract infection

EMQ 12: Dermatology

A   Hypertrophic scars
B   Acne vulgaris
C   Molluscum contagiosum
D   Atrophic scars
E   Wound healing
F   Keloid
H   Striae
I   Eczema
J   Acne rosacea
K   Warts
L   Fungal infections

For each statement below, select the appropriate diagnosis(es) from the list of options above. An option may be used once, more than once, or not at all. Up to four options may be used per case.

1   Is/are worse in adolescence

2   Cause(s) redness and itchiness of skin

3   Is/are worse in people who have more pigmented skins

4   Will not spontaneously regress or disappear

5   Is/are associated with significant morbidity

6   Swimming may worsen symptoms

7   Accounts for 90% of occupational skin problems

8   Complement is activated in the response

Answers and references

1: Being a doctor, being a patient

1.1　　(a) T　　(b) F　　(c) T　　(d) F　　(e) T

Offringa M, Moyer VA (2001) Evidence based paediatrics: Evidence-based management of seizures associated with fever. *Br Med J* **323**: 1111–4

1.2　　(a) F　　(b) T　　(c) T　　(d) T　　(e) F

Harnden A, Shakespeare J (2001) 10-minute consultation: MMR immunisation. *Br Med J* **323**: 32

1.3　　(a) F　　(b) F　　(c) F　　(d) F　　(e) F

Smith R. Clinical review: In search of 'non-disease'. *Br Med J* **324**: 883–5

1.4　　(a) T　　(b) F　　(c) T　　(d) F　　(e) T

Horrocks S, Anderson E, Salisbury C (2002) Systematic review of whether nurse practitioners working in primary care can provide equivalent care to doctors. *Br Med J* **324**: 819–23

1.5　　(a) T　　(b) F　　(c) T　　(d) F　　(e) F

Winkens R, Dinant G-J (2002) Evidence base of diagnostic research: Rational, cost effective use of investigations in clinical practice. *Br Med J* **324**: 783–5

1.6　　(a) F　　(b) T　　(c) T　　(d) F　　(e) F

Ellershaw J, Ward C (2003) Clinical review: Care of the dying patient: the last hours or days. *Br Med J* **326**: 30–4

1.7　　(a) T　　(b) T　　(c) F　　(d) F　　(e) T

Thwaites CL, Farrar JJ (2003) Preventing and treating tetanus. *Br Med J* **326**: 117–8

1.8　　(a) T　　(b) F　　(c) F　　(d) F　　(e) T

Elley CR, Kerse N, Arroll B, *et al* (2003) Effectiveness of counselling patients on physical activity in general practice: cluster randomised controlled trial. *Br Med J* **326**: 793–6

1.9　　(a) F　　(b) T　　(c) F　　(d) T　　(e) F

Grimwood K (2001) Legacy of bacterial meningitis in infancy. Br Med J 323: 523–4

British Medical Association (2003) *British National Formulary*. 46 edn. British Medical Association and Royal Pharmaceutical Society of Great Britain, London

1.10 (a) T (b) T (c) F (d) T (e) F
Snashall D (1996) ABC of work-related disorders: Hazards of work. *Br Med J* **313**: 161–3

1.11 (a) F (b) F (c) T (d) F (e) T
Fry J, ed (1982) *The Beecham Manual for Family Practice*. Section B3. MTP Press, Lancaster

1.12 (a) T (b) F (c) T (d) F (e) F
Knight B (1992) *Legal Aspects of Medical Practice*. Fifth edition. Churchill Livingstone,
   London

1.13 (a) T (b) F (c) T (d) T (e) T
Warrel DA, ed (2003) *Oxford Textbook of Medicine*. Fourth edition. Oxford University Press,
   Oxford

1.14 (a) F (b) F (c) T (d) T (e) T
Salisbury D, Begg N (1996) *Immunisation Against Infectious Disease*. The Stationery Office,
   London

1.15 (a) T (b) T (c) F (d) F (e) T
Warrel DA, ed (2003) *Oxford Textbook of Medicine*. Fourth edition. Oxford University Press,
   Oxford

1.16 (a) T (b) T (c) T (d) T (e) F
Warrel DA, ed (2003) *Oxford Textbook of Medicine*. Fourth edition. Oxford University Press,
   Oxford

1.17 (a) T (b) T (c) T (d) F (e) T
Rose G, Barker DJP (1983) *Epidemiology for the Uninitiated*. Third impression. British
   Medical Association, London

1.18 (a) F (b) F (c) T (d) F (e) F
Salisbury D, Begg N (1996) *Immunisation Against Infectious Disease*. The Stationery Office,
   London

1.19 (a) F (b) T (c) T (d) T (e) F
Knight B (1992) *Legal Aspects of Medical Practice*. Fifth edition. Churchill Livingstone,
   London

1.20   (a) T   (b) F   (c) T   (d) T   (e) T
Salisbury D, Begg N (1996) *Immunisation Against Infectious Disease*. The Stationery Office, London

2. Locomotion answers and references

2.1   (a) F   (b) F   (c) F   (d) T   (e) T
Dandy D, Edwards D (2003) *Essential Orthopaedics and Trauma*. Fourth edition. Churchill Livingston, London

2.2   (a) T   (b) F   (c) T   (d) T   (e) T
Yunus M, Aldag J (1996) Restless legs syndrome and leg cramps in fibromyalgia syndrome: a controlled study. *Br Med J* **312**: 1339

2.3   (a) T   (b) T   (c) F   (d) T   (e) T
Valman B, ed (2000) *ABC of One to Seven*. Fourth Edition. BMJ publications, London

2.4   (a) T   (b) T   (c) F   (d) T   (e) F
Hull D, Johnston D (1999) *Essential Paediatrics*. Fourth Edition. Churchill Livingston, London

2.5   (a) T   (b) F   (c) F   (d) T   (e) F
Hull D, Johnston D (1999) *Essential Paediatrics*. Fourth Edition. Churchill Livingston, London

2.6   (a) F   (b) T   (c) T   (d) T   (e) F
Speed CA (2001) Fortnightly review: Corticosteroid injections in tendon lesions. *Br Med J* **323**: 382–5

2.7   (a) T   (b) T   (c) F   (d) T   (e) T
Gillespie WJ (2001) Extracts from clinical evidence: Hip fracture. *Br Med J* **322**: 968–75

2.8   (a) T   (b) F   (c) F   (d) F   (e) F
Kendrick D, Fielding K, Bentley E *et al* (2001) Radiography of the lumbar spine in primary care patients with low back pain: randomised controlled trial. *Br Med J* **322**: 400–5

2.9   (a) T   (b) T   (c) F   (d) T   (e) F

Main CJ, Williams A (2002) ABC of psychological medicine: Musculoskeletal pain. *Br Med J*
325: 534–7

2.10   (a) F   (b) T   (c) F   (d) F   (e) T

Pal B (2002) 10-minute consultation: Paraesthesia. *Br Med J* **324**: 1501

2.11   (a) F   (b) T   (c) T   (d) F   (e) F

Bachmann LM, Kolb E, Koller MT *et al* (2003) Accuracy of Ottawa rules to exclude fractures
of the ankle and mid-foot: systematic review. *Br Med J* **326**: 417–9

2.12   (a) T   (b) T   (c) T   (d) T   (e) F

http://www.medicalprotection.org/medical/united_kingdom/publications/casebook/20_cauda.as
px (accessed 24 April 2003).

Shapiro S (2000) Medical realities of cauda equina syndrome secondary to lumbar disc
herniation. *Spine* **25**: 348–52

2.13   (a) T   (b) F   (c) F   (d) F   (e) T

Korthals-de Bos IBC, Hoving JL, van Tulder M *et al* (2003) Cost effectiveness of
physiotherapy, manual therapy, and general practitioner care for neck pain: economic
evaluation alongside a randomised controlled trial. Commentary: Bootstrapping simplifies
appreciation of statistical inferences. *Br Med J* **326**: 911

Van Tulder MW, Koes BW, Bouter LM (1997) Conservative treatment of acute and chronic
nonspecific low back pain: a systematic review of randomized controlled trials of the most
common interventions. *Spine* **22**: 2128–56

2.14   (a) F   (b) F   (c) T   (d) F   (e) F

McGill S (2002) *Low back disorders: evidence-based prevention and rehabilitation*. Human
Kinetics Europe Ltd, Leeds

Hutson M (2002) *Work Related Upper Limb Disorders: Recognition and Management*.
Churchill Livingston, London

2.15   (a) F   (b) T   (c) F   (d) T   (e) T

Marshall S. In: Godlee F, ed (2003) *Clinical Evidence Concise*. Issue nine. BMJ Publishing
Group, London: 220–2

2.16   (a) T   (b) T   (c) F   (d) F   (e) T

Warrel DA, ed (2003) *Oxford Textbook of Medicine*. Fourth edition. Oxford University Press,
Oxford

2.17   (a) F   (b) T   (c) T   (d) T   (e) F

Towheed TE, Anastassiades TP, Shea B *et al* (2001) Glucosamine therapy for treating osteoarthritis. In: The Cochrane Library. Issue 1. Update Software, Oxford

McAlindon TE, LaValley MP, Gulin JP *et al* (2000) Glucosamine and chondroitin for treatment of osteoarthritis. a systematic quality assessment and meta-analysis. *JAMA* **283**: 1469–75

Reginster JY, Deroisy R, Rovati LC *et al* (2001) Long-term effects of glucosamine sulphate on osteoarthritis progression: a randomised, placebo-controlled clinical trial. *Lancet* **357**: 251–6

Warrel DA, ed (2003) *Oxford Textbook of Medicine*. Fourth edition. Oxford University Press, Oxford

3. Blood and skin

3.1   (a) F   (b) T   (c) T   (d) T   (e) F

Crawford F, Hart R, Bell-Syer EM *et al* (2001) Extracts from 'Clinical Evidence': Athlete's foot and fungally infected toe nails. *Br Med J* **322**: 288–9

3.2   (a) T   (b) T   (c) F   (d) T   (e) T

Schoonhoven L, Haalboom JRE, Bousema MT *et al* for the prePURSE study group (2002) Prospective cohort study of routine use of risk assessment scales for prediction of pressure ulcers. *Br Med J* **325**: 797–800

3.3   (a) T   (b) F   (c) T   (d) T   (e) F

Regan F, Taylor C (2002) Recent developments: Blood transfusion medicine. *Br Med J* **325**: 143–7

3.4   (a) F   (b) T   (c) T   (d) T   (e) F

Barnetson R StC, Rogers M (2002) Clinical review: Childhood atopic eczema. *Br Med J* **324**: 1376–9

3.5   (a) T   (b) F   (c) T   (d) F   (e) T

Harding KG, Morris HL, Patel GK (2002) Science, medicine, and the future: Healing chronic wounds. *Br Med J* **324**: 160–3

3.6   (a) F   (b) T   (c) F   (d) F   (e) F

Bayat A, McGrouther DA, Ferguson MJW (2003) Clinical review: Skin scarring. *Br Med J* **326**: 88–92

3.7   (a) T   (b) F   (c) F   (d) F   (e) F

Fry A, Verne J (2003) Preventing skin cancer. *Br Med J* **326**: 114–5

3.8   (a) T   (b) F   (c) F   (d) T   (e) F

Fuller LC, Child FJ, Midgley G *et al* (2003) Clinical review: Diagnosis and management of scalp ringworm. *Br Med J* **326**: 539–41

3.9   (a) F   (b) T   (c) F   (d) T   (e) T

Johnson RW, Dworkin RH (2003) Clinical review: Treatment of herpes zoster and postherpetic neuralgia. *Br Med J* **326**: 748–50

3.10   (a) T   (b) T   (c) T   (d) T   (e) F

Goddard AF, McIntyre AS, Scott BB (2000) Guidelines for the management of iron deficiency anaemia. British Society of Gastroenterology. *Gut* **46** Suppl 3-4: IV1–IV5

3.11   (a) F   (b) T   (c) T   (d) T   (e) F

Liesner RJ, Goldstone AH (1997) ABC of clinical haematology: The acute leukaemias. *Br Med J* **314**: 733

3.12   (a) F   (b) F   (c) F   (d) T   (e) T

Hunter J, Savin J, Dahl M (2002) *Clinical Dermatology*. Third edition. Blackwell, Oxford

3.13   (a) T   (b) T   (c) F   (d) F   (e) T

Hunter J, Savin J, Dahl M (2002) *Clinical Dermatology*. Third edition. Blackwell, Oxford

3.14   (a) T   (b) F   (c) T   (d) T   (e) T

Kirby DT (2002) In: Kumar P, Clark M, eds. *Clinical Medicine*. Fifth edition. Ballière Tindall, London

3.15   (a) F   (b) F   (c) F   (d) T   (e) T

Fuller LC, Child FJ, Midgley G, *et al* (2003) Clinical review: Diagnosis and management of scalp ringworm. *Br Med J* **326**: 539–41

3.16   (a) F   (b) T   (c) T   (d) F   (e) T

Lydyard PM, Lakhani SR, Dogan A, *et al* (2000) *Pathology Integrated: an A–Z of Disease and its Pathogenesis*. Arnold, London: 53–4

4. Circulation

4.1   (a) T   (b) F   (c) T   (d) T   (e) F
Straus SE (2001) Recent advances: Geriatric medicine. *Br Med J* **322**: 86–9

4.2   (a) F   (b) T   (c) T   (d) F   (e) T
Padwal R, Straus SE, McAlister FA (2001) Evidence based management of hypertension:
    Cardiovascular risk factors and their effects on the decision to treat hypertension: evidence
    based review. *Br Med J* **322**: 977–80

4.3   (a) F   (b) T   (c) T   (d) F   (e) T
Turpie AGG, Chin BSP, Lip GYH (2002) ABC of antithrombotic therapy: Venous
    thromboembolism: pathophysiology, clinical features, and prevention. *Br Med J* **325**:
    887–90

4.4   (a) T   (b) F   (c) T   (d) F   (e) F
Lip GYH, Kamath S, Hart RG (2002) ABC of antithrombotic therapy: Antithrombotic therapy
    for cerebrovascular disorders. *Br Med J* **325**: 1161–3

4.5   (a) T   (b) F   (c) T   (d) T   (e) T
Bosch J, Yusuf S, Pogue J, *et al* (2002) Use of ramipril in preventing stroke: double blind
    randomised trial. *Br Med J* **324**: 699–702

4.6   (a) T   (b) F   (c) F   (d) F   (e) F
Lip GYH, Hart RG, Conway DSG (2002) ABC of antithrombotic therapy: Antithrombotic
    therapy for atrial fibrillation. *Br Med J* **325**: 1022–5

4.7   (a) T   (b) F   (c) F   (d) T   (e) T
Blann AD, Landray MJ, Lip GYH (2002) ABC of antithrombotic therapy: An overview of
    antithrombotic therapy. *Br Med J* **325**: 762–5

4.8   (a) T   (b) F   (c) F   (d) T   (e) T
Cowie MR, Zaphiriou A (2002) Recent developments: Management of chronic heart failure. *Br
    Med J* **325**: 422–5

4.9   (a) F   (b) T   (c) F   (d) F   (e) T
A'Court C (2002) 10-minute consultation: Newly diagnosed hypertension. *Br Med J* **324**: 1375

4.10   (a) T   (b) T   (c) F   (d) T   (e) T
Williams B (2003) Drug treatment of hypertension. *Br Med J* **326**: 61–2

4.11   (a) F   (b) T   (c) T   (d) F   (e) F
Slovis C, Jenkins R (2002) ABC of clinical electrocardiography: Conditions not primarily affecting the heart. *Br Med J* **324**: 1320–3

4.12   (a) T   (b) T   (c) T   (d) T   (e) T
Hill J, Timmis A (2002) ABC of clinical electrocardiography: Exercise tolerance testing. *Br Med J* **324**: 1084

4.13   (a) F   (b) T   (c) F   (d) T   (e) F
Channer K, Morris F (2002) ABC of clinical electrocardiography: Myocardial ischaemia. *Br Med J* **324**: 1023–6

4.14   (a) F   (b) F   (c) F   (d) T   (e) T
Goodacre S, Irons R (2002) ABC of clinical electrocardiography: Atrial arrhythmias. *Br Med J* **324**: 594–7

4.15   (a) F   (b) F   (c) T   (d) T   (e) T
Da Costa D, Brady WJ, Edhouse J (2002) ABC of clinical electrocardiography: Bradycardias and atrioventricular conduction block. *Br Med J* **324**: 535–8

4.16   (a) T   (b) F   (c) F   (d) T   (e) F
Blann AD, Fitzmaurice DA, Lip GYH (2003) ABC of antithrombotic therapy: Anticoagulation in hospitals and general practice. *Br Med J* **326**: 153–6

4.17   (a) T   (b) F   (c) F   (d) F   (e) F
Burns P, Gough S, Bradbury AW (2003) Clinical review: Management of peripheral arterial disease in primary care. *Br Med J* **326**: 584–8

4.18   (a) T   (b) F   (c) F   (d) F   (e) F
Morris F, Brady WJ (2002) ABC of clinical electrocardiography: Acute myocardial infarction-Part I. *Br Med J* **324**: 831–4

4.19   (a) T   (b) T   (c) F   (d) F   (e) T
Meek S, Morris F (2002) ABC of clinical electrocardiography: Introduction. I-Leads, rate, rhythm, and cardiac axis. *Br Med J* **324**: 415–8

4.20 (a) F (b) F (c) F (d) T (e) T

British Medical Association (2003) *British National Formulary*. 46 edn. British Medical
Association and Royal Pharmaceutical Society of Great Britain, London

4.21 (a) F (b) T (c) F (d) T (e) T

Prendergast B (2002) Diagnosis of infective endocarditis. *Br Med J* **325**: 845–6

5. Respiration

5.1 (a) F (b) T (c) T (d) T (e) F

Cates C (2001) Extracts from 'Clinical Evidence': Chronic asthma. *Br Med J* **323**: 976–9

5.2 (a) F (b) F (c) T (d) F (e) F

Kerstjens HAM, Groen HJ, van der Bij W (2001) Recent advances: Respiratory medicine. *Br
Med J* **323**: 1349–53

5.3 (a) F (b) F (c) F (d) F (e) F

Keeley D (2002) Guidelines for managing community acquired pneumonia in adults. *Br Med J*
324: 436–7

5.4 (a) F (b) T (c) F (d) T (e) F

The British Thoracic Society/Scottish Intercollegiate Guideline Network (2003) British
guideline on the management of asthma. *Thorax* **58**(S1): i1–i94.

5.5 (a) T (b) T (c) T (d) F (e) F

Warrel DA, ed (2003) *Oxford Textbook of Medicine*. Fourth edition. Oxford University Press,
Oxford

5.6 (a) T (b) T (c) F (d) T (e) F

Reece J, Price J, eds (2000) *ABC of Asthma*. Fourth edition. BMJ Books, London

5.7 (a) F (b) T (c) F (d) T (e) T

Kumar PJ, Clark ML, eds (2002) *Clinical Medicine*. Fifth edition. Saunders, London

5.8 (a) F (b) T (c) T (d) F (e) F

Stout JE, Yu VL, Muraca P, *et al* (1992) Potable water as a cause of sporadic cases of
community-acquired legionnaires' disease. *N Engl J Med* **326**: 151–5

5.9   (a) T   (b) F   (c) T   (d) F   (e) T

British Thoracic Society (1997) Guidelines on the management of COPD. *Thorax* **52**: 5

5.10   (a) T   (b) F   (c) F   (d) T   (e) T

Reece J, Price J, eds (2000) *ABC of Asthma*. Fourth edition. BMJ Books, London

5.11   (a) F   (b) T   (c) T   (d) T   (e) T

Lydyard P, Lakhani S, Dogan A *et al* (2000) Pathology Integrated. Arnold, London

BNF 46 (2003) British National Formulary. Forty sixth edition. British Medical Association
    and Royal Pharmaceutical Society of Great Britain, London

5.12   (a) T   (b) F   (c) T   (d) F   (e) F

Singh S, Madge S, Lipman M (2002) Tuberculosis in primary care. *Br J Gen Pract* **52**: 357–8

5.13   (a) F   (b) T   (c) T   (d) T   (e) F

Hopcroft K, Forte (2003) *Symptom sorter*. Second edition. Radcliffe Medical Press, Oxford

5.14   (a) T   (b) F   (c) T   (d) T   (e) F

Warrel DA, ed (2003) *Oxford Textbook of Medicine*. Fourth edition. Oxford University Press,
    Oxford

5.15   (a) T   (b) F   (c) T   (d) F   (e) T

Cornford CS (2000) Lay beliefs of patients using domiciliary oxygen: a qualitative study from
    general practice. *Br J Gen Pract* **50**: 791–3

5.16   (a) T   (b) T   (c) T   (d) T   (e) T

Meredith SK, Taylor VM, McDonald JC (1991) Occupational respiratory disease in the United
    Kingdom 1989: a report to the British Thoracic Society and the Society of Occupational
    Medicine by the SWORD project group. *Br J Industrial Med* **48**: 292–8

5.17   (a) T   (b) T   (c) F   (d) T   (e) F

Holmes WF, Macfarlane JT, Macfarlane RM, *et al* (2001) Symptoms, signs, and prescribing
    for acute lower respiratory tract illness. *Br J Gen Pract* **51**: 177–81

5.18   (a) T   (b) T   (c) T   (d) T   (e) T

Hay AD, Wilson A (2002) The natural history of acute cough in children aged 0 to 4 years in
    primary care: a systematic review. *Br J Gen Pract* **52**: 401–9

5.19   (a) F   (b) F   (c) T   (d) T   (e) F
Hopcroft K, Forte (2003) *Symptom sorter*. Second edition. Radcliffe Medical Press, Oxford

5.20   (a) T   (b) T   (c) F   (d) F   (e) F
Warrel DA, ed (2003) *Oxford Textbook of Medicine*. Fourth edition. Oxford University Press, Oxford

6. Homeostasis and hormones

6.1   (a) T   (b) F   (c) F   (d) T   (e) T
Barry MJ, Roehrborn CG (2001) Extracts from 'Clinical Evidence': Benign prostatic hyperplasia. *Br Med J* **323**: 1042–6

6.2   (a) F   (b) T   (c) F   (d) T   (e) T
Gennari FJ (1998) Current concepts: Hypokalemia. *N Engl J Med* **339**: 451–8

6.3   (a) T   (b) T   (c) F   (d) T   (e) F
Haslett C, Savill J (2001) Why is apoptosis important to clinicians? *Br Med J* **322**: 1499–1500
Lin J-D (2001) The role of apoptosis in autoimmune thyroid disorders and thyroid cancer. *Br Med J* **322**: 1525–32
Renehan AG, Booth C, Potten CS (2001) What is apoptosis, and why is it important? *Br Med J* **322**: 1536–40

6.4   (a) T   (b) F   (c) T   (d) T   (e) F
Powell P, Bentall RP, Nye FJ *et al* (2001) Randomised controlled trial of patient education to encourage graded exercise in chronic fatigue syndrome. *Br Med J* **322**: 387–90

6.5   (a) T   (b) F   (c) T   (d) F   (e) T
Dearnaley DP, Huddart RA, Horwich A (2001) Regular review: Managing testicular cancer. *Br Med J* **322**: 1583–8

6.6   (a) T   (b) F   (c) F   (d) F   (e) T
McGovern MC, Glasgow JFT, Stewart MC (2001) Lesson of the week: Reye's syndrome and aspirin: lest we forget. *Br Med J* **322**: 1591–2

6.7   (a) T   (b) T   (c) F   (d) F   (e) F
Sanderson RJ, Ironside JAD (2002) Clinical review: Squamous carcinomas of the head and neck. *Br Med J* **325**: 822–7

6.8   (a) T   (b) T   (c) F   (d) F   (e) F

Wright PJ, English PJ, Hungin APS *et al* (2002) Managing acute renal colic across the primary-secondary care interface: a pathway of care based on evidence and consensus. *Br Med J* **325**: 1408–12

6.9   (a) T   (b) F   (c) T   (d) F   (e) T

Ward K, Hilton P on behalf of the United Kingdom and Ireland Tension-free vaginal Tape Trial Group (2002) Prospective multicentre randomised trial of tension-free vaginal tape and colposuspension for stress incontinence. *Br Med J* **325**: 67–70

6.10   (a) T   (b) F   (c) F   (d) F   (e) F

Parmar MS (2002) Clinical review: Chronic renal disease. *Br Med J* **325**: 85–90

6.11   (a) T   (b) T   (c) T   (d) F   (e) F

Andrews PA (2002) Recent developments: Renal transplantation. *Br Med J* **324**: 530–4

6.12   (a) F   (b) T   (c) F   (d) T   (e) F

Jones GC, Macklin JP, Alexander WD (2003) Contraindications to the use of metformin. *Br Med J* **326** :4–5

6.13   (a) F   (b) T   (c) F   (d) T   (e) T

Toft AD, Beckett GJ (2003) Thyroid function tests and hypothyroidism. *Br Med J* **326**: 295–6

6.14   (a) F   (b) T   (c) F   (d) F   (e) F

Hall G, Patel P, Protheroe A (1998) Key Topics in Oncology. Abingdon: Bios.
Lindblom A, Liljegren A (2000) Tumour markers in malignancies. *Br Med J* **320**: 424–7

6.15   (a) T   (b) T   (c) F   (d) F   (e) T

Leibovici L (2002) Antibiotic treatment for cystitis. *Br J Gen P* 52: 708–10

7. The 'Senses'

7.1   (a) T   (b) F   (c) T   (d) T   (e) F

Schrader H, Stovner LJ, Helde G *et al* (2001) Prophylactic treatment of migraine with angiotensin inhibitor (lisinopril): randomised, placebo controlled, crossover study. *Br Med J* **322**: 19–22

7.2 (a) T (b) T (c) F (d) T (e) F

Wong TY (2001) Regular review: Effect of increasing age on cataract surgery outcomes in the very elderly. *Br Med J* **322**: 1104–6

7.3 (a) T (b) T (c) T (d) F (e) T

Little P, Gould C, Williamson I *et al* (2001) Pragmatic randomised controlled trial of two prescribing strategies for childhood otitis media. *Br Med J* **322**: 336–42

7.4 (a) T (b) F (c) T (d) T (e) T

Steiner TJ, Fontebasso M (2002) Clinical review: Headache. *Br Med J* 325: 881–6

7.5 (a) T (b) T (c) T (d) F (e) T

Acuin J (2002) Extracts from Concise Clinical Evidence: Chronic suppurative otitis media. *Br Med J* **325**: 1159–60

7.6 (a) F (b) T (c) T (d) T (e) T

Fredrick DR (2002) Clinical review: Myopia. *Br Med J* **324**: 11950–9

7.7 (a) T (b) F (c) F (d) F (e) F

Chopdar A, Chakravarthy U, Verma D (2003) Clinical review: Age related macular degeneration. *Br Med J* **326**: 485–8

7.8 (a) T (b) F (c) F (d) T (e) F

O'Neill P (1999) Clinical review: Acute otitis media. *Br Med J* **319**: 833–5

7.9 (a) T (b) F (c) T (d) F (e) T

Fisher M (1995) Fortnightly review: Treatment of acute anaphylaxis. *Br Med J* **311**: 731–3.
Sanderson RJ, Ironside JAD (2002) Squamous cell carcinomas of the head and neck. *Br Med J* **325**: 822–7

7.10 (a) T (b) T (c) T (d) T (e) F

Sowka JW, Kabat AG *Double trouble: how to diagnose diplopia. Review of Optometry OnLine* July 15, available online: http://www.revoptom.com/archive/features/ro0700f7.htm (accessed 24 Apr 2003)

7.11 (a) F (b) T (c) F (d) T (e) T

Lempert T, Gresty MA, Bronstein AM (1995) Benign positional vertigo: recognition and treatment. *Br Med J* **311**: 489–91

Saeed SR (1998) Fortnightly review: Diagnosis and treatment of Ménière's disease. *Br Med J*
316: 368–72

7.12   (a) F   (b) T   (c) T   (d) T   (e) F

Carding P, Wade A (2000) Managing dysphonia caused by misuse and overuse. *Br Med J*
321:1544–5

Wilson J, Deary I, Scott S *et al* (1995) Functional dysphonia. *Br Med J* **311**: 1039–40

7.13   (a) T   (b) F   (c) T   (d) F   (e) T

British Medical Association (2003) *British National Formulary*. 46 edn. British Medical
Association and Royal Pharmaceutical Society of Great Britain, London

Sowka JW, Gurwood AS, Kabat AG Handbook of Ocular Disease Management, available
online: http://www.revoptom.com/handbook/ (accessed 20 Sept 2003)

Tepper S Drug (2000) Interactions and the triptans. *Primary Care Special Edition* **5** (2):
31–4http://mcmahonmed.com/se/pc/pdf/triptans.pdf (accessed 20 Sept 2003)

7.14   (a) T   (b) F   (c) T   (d) F   (e) F

Tanner K, Fitzsimmons G, Carrol ED *et al* (2002) Lesson of the week: Haemophilus
influenzae type b epiglottitis as a cause of acute upper airways obstruction in children. *Br
Med J* **325**: 1099–100

7.15   (a) T   (b) T   (c) T   (d) F   (e) T

Russ S (2001) Measuring the prevalence of permanent childhood hearing impairment. *Br Med
J* **323**: 525–6

Fortnum HM, Summerfield AQ, Marshall DH *et al* (2001) Prevalence of permanent childhood
hearing impairment in the United Kingdom and implications for universal neonatal
hearing screening: questionnaire-based ascertainment study. *Br Med J* **323**: 536–40

8. Digestion and nutrition

8.1   (a) T   (b) F   (c) F   (d) F   (e) T

Beckingham IJ, Ryder SD (2001) ABC of diseases of liver, pancreas, and biliary system:
Investigation of liver and biliary disease. *Br Med J* **322**: 33–6

8.2   (a) T   (b) F   (c) T   (d) F   (e) T

Edmunds L, Waters E, Elliott EJ (2001) Evidence-based paediatrics: Evidence-based
management of childhood obesity. *Br Med J* **323**: 916–9

8.3   (a) T   (b) F   (c) T   (d) F   (e) T
Owen W (2001) ABC of the upper gastrointestinal tract: Dysphagia. *Br Med J* **323**: 850–3

8.4   (a) F   (b) T   (c) T   (d) T   (e) F
Bowles MJ, Benjamin IS (2001) ABC of the upper gastrointestinal tract: Cancer of the
  stomach and pancreas *Br Med J* **323**: 1413–6

8.5   (a) T   (b) F   (c) T   (d) F   (e) T
Talley NJ, Phung N, Kalantar JS (2001) ABC of the upper gastrointestinal tract. Indigestion:
  When is it functional? *Br Med J* **323**: 1294–7

8.6   (a) T   (b) T   (c) F   (d) F   (e) T
Krige JEJ, Beckingham IJ (2001) ABC of diseases liver, pancreas, and biliary system: Portal
  hypertension-2. Ascites, encephalopathy, and other conditions. *Br Med J* **322**: 416–8

8.7   (a) F   (b) T   (c) T   (d) T   (e) T
Sherwood P, Lyburn I, Brown S *et al* (2001) How are abnormal results for liver function tests
  dealt with in primary care? Audit of yield and impact. *Br Med J* **322**: 276–8

8.8   (a) T   (b) F   (c) T   (d) T   (e) F
Noël PH, Pugh JA (2002) Clinical review: Management of overweight and obese adults. *Br
  Med J* **325**: 757–61

8.9   (a) T   (b) F   (c) T   (d) F   (e) F
Jankowski J, Jones R, Delaney B *et al* (2002) 10-minute consultation: Gastro-oesophageal
  reflux disease. *Br Med J* **325**: 945

8.10   (a) T   (b) F   (c) T   (d) F   (e) F
Guthrie E, Thompson D (2002) ABC of psychological medicine: Abdominal pain and
  functional gastrointestinal disorders. *Br Med J* **325**: 701–3

8.11   (a) T   (b) F   (c) F   (d) T   (e) T
Elliott R, Ong TJ (2002) Science, medicine, and the future: Nutritional genomics. *Br Med J*
  324: 1438–42

8.12   (a) F   (b) F   (c) T   (d) F   (e) T
Hall G, Patel P, Protheroe A (1998) *Key Topics in Oncology*. Bios, London

8.13　(a) F　(b) F　(c) T　(d) T　(e) F

Department of Health (2001) *Health Information for Overseas Travel*. DOH, London

British Medical Association (2003) *British National Formulary*. 46 edn. British Medical
　　Association and Royal Pharmaceutical Society of Great Britain, London

8.14　(a) F　(b) T　(c) T　(d) T　(e) F

Valman B, ed (2000) *ABC of One to Seven*. Fourth edition. BMJ Publications, London

8.15　(a) F　(b) T　(c) T　(d) F　(e) T

Warrel DA, ed (2003) *Oxford Textbook of Medicine*. Fourth edition. Oxford University Press,
　　Oxford

8.16　(a) F　(b) T　(c) T　(d) F　(e) T

Warrel DA, ed (2003) *Oxford Textbook of Medicine*. Fourth edition. Oxford University Press,
　　Oxford

8.17　(a) T　(b) F　(c) T　(d) F　(e) T

Warrel DA, ed (2003) *Oxford Textbook of Medicine*. Fourth edition. Oxford University Press,
　　Oxford

8.18　(a) T　(b) T　(c) F　(d) T　(e) F

Hull D, Johnston D (1999) *Essential Paediatrics*. Fourth edition. Churchill Livingstone,
　　Edinburgh

8.19　(a) T　(b) T　(c) F　(d) T　(e) T

Maria G, Cassetta E, Gui D *et al* (1998) A comparison of botulinum toxin and saline for the
　　treatment of chronic anal fissure. *New Engl J Med* **338**: 217–20

Madoff R (1998) Pharmacologic therapy for anal fissure. *New Engl J Med* **338**: 257–9

8.20　(a) F　(b) T　(c) F　(d) T　(e) T

Kumar PJ, Clark ML, eds (2002) *Clinical Medicine*. Fifth edition. Saunders, London

8.21　(a) T　(b) F　(c) T　(d) T　(e) T

Hull D, Johnston D (1999) *Essential Paediatrics*. Fourth edition. Churchill Livingstone,
　　Edinburgh

8.22   (a) F   (b) T   (c) T   (d) T   (e) F

British Medical Association (2003) *British National Formulary*. 46 edn. British Medical
   Association and Royal Pharmaceutical Society of Great Britain, London

9. Reproduction

9.1   (a) T   (b) T   (c) F   (d) T   (e) T

Gilson R, Mindel A (2001) Sexually transmitted diseases. *Br Med J* **322**: 1160–4

9.2   (a) F   (b) F   (c) T   (d) T   (e) T

British Medical Association (2003) *British National Formulary*. 46 edn. British Medical
   Association and Royal Pharmaceutical Society of Great Britain, London
Glasier A, Gebbie A, Loudon N (2000) *Handbook of Family Planning and Reproductive
   Healthcare*. Fourth edition. Churchill Livingstone, London

9.3   (a) T   (b) T   (c) T   (d) F   (e) F

Grant AD, De Cock KM (2001) ABC of AIDS: HIV infection and AIDS in the developing
   world. *Br Med J* **322**: 1475–8

9.4   (a) T   (b) F   (c) F   (d) F   (e) T

Ankum WM, Wieringa-de Waard M, Bindels PJE (2001) Regular review: Management of
   spontaneous miscarriage in the first trimester: an example of putting informed decision
   making into practice. *Br Med J* **322**: 1343–6

9.5   (a) F   (b) T   (c) T   (d) T   (e) T

Ross J (2001) Extracts from Clinical Evidence: Pelvic inflammatory disease. *Br Med J* **322**:
   658–9

9.6   (a) T   (b) T   (c) T   (d) F   (e) F

Fender GRK, Prentice A, Nixon RM *et al* (2001) Management of menorrhagia: an audit of
   practices in East Anglia menorrhagia education study. *Br Med J* **322**: 523–4

9.7   (a) F   (b) T   (c) T   (d) F   (e) T

Duley L, Henderson-Smart D, Knight M *et al* (2001) Antiplatelet drugs for prevention of pre-
   eclampsia and its consequences: systematic review. *Br Med J* **322**: 329–33

9.8   (a) T   (b) F   (c) T   (d) T   (e) F

Prentice A (2001) Regular review: Endometriosis. *Br Med J* **323**: 93–5

9.9 (a) T (b) F (c) T (d) F (e) T

Marrazzo J (2002) Extracts from Concise Clinical Evidence: Vulvovaginal candidiasis. *Br Med J* **325**: 586

9.10 (a) T (b) T (c) F (d) T (e) F

Cahill DJ, Wardle PG (2002) Clinical review: Management of infertility. *Br Med J* **325**: 28–32

9.11 (a) T (b) T (c) F (d) F (e) T

DiCenso A, Guyatt G, Willan A *et al* (2002) Interventions to reduce unintended pregnancies among adolescents: systematic review of randomised controlled trials. *Br Med J* **324**: 1426–30

9.12 (a) F (b) F (c) T (d) F (e) T

Thakar R, Stanton S (2002) Regular review: Management of genital prolapse. *Br Med J* **324**: 1258–62

9.13 (a) F (b) T (c) T (d) F (e) F

Morrow M, Gradishar W (2002) Recent developments: Breast cancer. *Br Med J* **324**: 410–4

9.14 (a) T (b) F (c) F (d) T (e) T

McIntyre J, Gray G (2002) What can we do to reduce mother to child transmission of HIV? *Br Med J* **24**: 218–21

9.15 (a) F (b) F (c) T (d) T (e) F

Rymer J, Wilson R, Ballard K (2003) Clinical review: making decisions about hormone replacement therapy. *Br Med J* **326**: 322–6

9.16 (a) T (b) T (c) T (d) F (e) F

Enkin M, Keirse M, Renfrew M *et al* (2000) A Guide to Effective Care in Pregnancy and Childbirth. Third edition. Oxford University Press, Oxford

9.17 (a) F (b) F (c) T (d) F (e) T

Guillebaud J (1995) *Contraception—Your Questions Answered*. Third edition. Churchill Livingstone, London

9.18 (a) T (b) F (c) T (d) T (e) F

Enkin M, Keirse M, Renfrew M *et al* (2000) *A Guide to Effective Care in Pregnancy and Childbirth*. Third edition. Oxford University Press, Oxford

9.19   (a) T   (b) F   (c) T   (d) T   (e) F

MacKinnon M (2002) *Providing Diabetes Care in General Practice*. Fourth edition. Class
   Publishing, London

10. Growth and development

10.1   (a) T   (b) T   (c) T   (d) F   (e) F

Wade S, Kilgour T (2001) Extracts from Clinical Evidence: Infantile colic. *Br Med J* **323**:
   437–40

10.2   (a) T   (b) F   (c) F   (d) F   (e) T

Evans JHC (2001) Evidence-based paediatrics: Evidence-based management of nocturnal
   enuresis. *Br Med J* **323**: 1167–9

10.3   (a) T   (b) F   (c) F   (d) T   (e) T

Saenger P (1996) Current concepts: Turner's syndrome. *New Engl J Med* **335**: 1749–54

10.4   (a) F   (b) F   (c) F   (d) F   (e) T

Valman B, ed (2000) *ABC of One to Seven*. Fourth edition. BMJ publications, London

10.5   (a) F   (b) T   (c) F   (d) T   (e) F

Valman B, ed (2000) *ABC of One to Seven*. Fourth edition. BMJ publications, London

10.6   (a) F   (b) T   (c) F   (d) T   (e) T

Hull D, Johnston D (1999) *Essential Paediatrics*. Fourth edition. Churchill Livingstone,
   London

10.7   (a) T   (b) T   (c) T   (d) F   (e) F

Valman B, ed (2000) *ABC of One to Seven*. Fourth edition. BMJ publications, London

10.8   (a) F   (b) T   (c) F   (d) T   (e) F

Illingworth R (1991) *Basic Developmental Screening 0–4 years*. Fifth edition. Blackwell
   Books, Oxford

10.9   (a) F   (b) F   (c) F   (d) F   (e) T

Enkin M, Keirse M, Renfrew M *et al* (2000) *A Guide to Effective Care in Pregnancy and
   Childbirth*. Third edition. Oxford University Press, Oxford

10.10 (a) F (b) F (c) F (d) F (e) T
Eliason BC, Lewan RB (1998) Gastroenteritis in children: principles of diagnosis and treatment. *Am Fam Phy* **1115**: 1–11

10.11 (a) T (b) F (c) T (d) T (e) F
American Academy of Pediatrics Committee on Newborn (1996) *Pediatrics* **98**:141–2

10.12 (a) F (b) F (c) T (d) T (e) T
Hippisley-Cox J, Groom L, Kendrick D *et al* (2002) Cross sectional survey of socioeconomic variations in severity and mechanism of childhood injuries in Trent 1992–7. *Br Med J* **324**: 1132–4
Halman SI, Chipman M, Parkin PC *et al* (2002) Are seat belt restraints as effective in school age children as in adults? *Br Med J* **324**: 1123–4

10.13 (a) F (b) F (c) T (d) T (e) T
Aicardi J (1998) The aetiology of developmental delay. *Seminars in Paediatric Neurology* **5**: 15–20

10.14 (a) T (b) F (c) T (d) T (e) T
Leung AK, Sigalet DL (2003) Acute abdominal pain in children. *Am Fam Phy* **67**: 2321–6
Mapagu C, Lam A, Martin C *et al* (2003) Intermittent intussusception. *J Paediatr Child Health* **39**: 147–8

10.15 (a) T (b) T (c) F (d) F (e) T
Fortnum HM, Summerfield AQ, Marshall DH *et al* (2001) Prevalence of permanent childhood hearing impairment in the United Kingdom and implications for universal neonatal hearing screening: questionnaire based ascertainment study. *Br Med J* **323**: 536–40

10.16 (a) T (b) F (c) T (d) T (e) T
Royal College of Ophthalmologists (2000) *Guidelines for the Management of Strabismus and Amblyopia in Childhood*. RCO, London

10.17 (a) T (b) F (c) T (d) T (e) T
Yule W, Rutter M (1987) *Language Development and Disorders*. Cambridge University Press, Cambridge

10.18 (a) T (b) T (c) T (d) T (e) T
Hull D, Johnston D (1999) *Essential Paediatrics*. Fourth edition. Churchill Livingstone, London

10.19 (a) F (b) T (c) F (d) F (e) F
Seymour CA, Thomason MJ, Chalmers RA *et al* (1997) Neonatal screening for inborn errors of metabolism: a systematic review. *Health Technol Assess* **1** (i–iv): 1–95

10.20 (a) F (b) T (c) F (d) F (e) F
Hull D, Johnston D (1999) *Essential Paediatrics*. Fourth edition. Churchill Livingstone, London

11. The mind

11.1 (a) T (b) T (c) F (d) T (e) F
Isacsson G, Rich CI (2001) Regular review: Management of patients who deliberately harm themselves. *Br Med J* **322**: 213–5

11.2 (a) T (b) F (c) F (d) T (e) F
Hay PJ, Bacaltchuk J (2001) Extracts from Clinical Evidence: Bulimia nervosa. *Br Med J* **323**: 33–7

11.3 (a) T (b) T (c) T (d) F (e) T
Bass C, Mayou R (2002) ABC of psychological medicine: Chest pain. *Br Med J* **325**: 588–91

11.4 (a) T (b) T (c) F (d) F (e) T
House A, Stark D (2002) ABC of psychological medicine: Anxiety in medical patients. *Br Med J* **325**: 207–9

11.5 (a) T (b) F (c) T (d) F (e) T
Peveler R, Carson A, Rodin G (2002) ABC of psychological medicine: Depression in medical patients. *Br Med J* **325**: 149–52

11.6 (a) T (b) F (c) F (d) T (e) F
Small GW. Clinical review: What we need to know about age related memory loss. *Br Med J* **324**: 1502–5

11.7 (a) F (b) T (c) F (d) T (e) F
Dinan TG (2002) Lithium in bipolar mood disorder. *Br Med J* **324**: 989–90

11.8   (a) T   (b) F   (c) F   (d) T   (e) F
Cutler NR, Post RM, Rey A *et al* (1981) Depression-dependent dyskinesias in two cases of
    manic-depressive illness. *New Eng J Med* **04**: 1088–9

11.9   (a) T   (b) T   (c) F   (d) T   (e) F
Szatmari P (2003) The causes of autism spectrum disorders. *Br Med J* **326**: 173–4

11.10   (a) F   (b) F   (c) T   (d) F   (e) T
Bhui K, Weich S, Lloyd K (1998) *Pocket Psychiatry*. Third edition. Saunders, London

11.11   (a) F   (b) T   (c) T   (d) F   (e) T
Hultman C, Sparén P, Takei N *et al* Prenatal and perinatal risk factors for schizophrenia,
    affective psychosis, and reactive psychosis of early onset: case-control study. *Br Med J*
    318: 421–6
Zammit S, Allebeck P, Andreasson S *et al* (2002) Self-reported cannabis use as a risk factor for
    schizophrenia in Swedish conscripts of 1969: historical cohort study. *Br Med J* **325**: 1199

11.12   (a) T   (b) F   (c) F   (d) F   (e) T
Notcutt W, Healey A, Ashton J *et al* (2000) Improving the debate on cannabis. *Br Med J* **320**:
    1671
Patton G, Coffey C, Carlin J, *et al* (2002) Cannabis use and mental health in young people:
    cohort study. *Br Med J* **325**: 1195–8

11.13   (a) T   (b) F   (c) F   (d) T   (e) T
Hallstrom C, McClure N (2000) Anxiety and Depression — Your Questions Answered.
    Churchill Livingstone, London

11.14   (a) T   (b) F   (c) T   (d) T   (e) F
Ashworth M, Gerada C (1997) ABC of mental health: Addiction and dependence II: Alcohol.
    Br Med J **315**: 358–60

11.15   (a) T   (b) T   (c) F   (d) F   (e) T
Bhui K, Weich S, Lloyd K (1998) *Pocket Psychiatry*. Third edition. WB Saunders, London

11.16   (a) T   (b) T   (c) T   (d) F   (e) T
Gerada C, Ashworth M (1997) ABC of mental health: Addiction and dependence I: Illicit
    drugs. *Br Med J* **315**: 297–300

11.17 (a) T   (b) F   (c) T   (d) F   (e) T

Online at: http://www.intellectualdisability.info/main.html, St Georges Hospital Medical
    School (accessed 24 April 2003)

11.18 (a) T   (b) F   (c) F   (d) F   (e) T

Burton C (2003) Beyond somatisation: a review of the understanding and treatment of
    medically explained symptoms. *Br J Gen Prac* **53**: 595–8

11.19 (a) F   (b) F   (c) F   (d) F   (e) T

Thapar AK, Thapar A (2003) Attention deficit hyperactivity disorder. *Br J Gen Prac* **53**:
    225–30

12. Emergency medicine

12.1 (a) F   (b) F   (c) T   (d) T   (e) T

Evison D, Hinsley D, Rice P (2002) Regular review: Chemical weapons. *Br Med J* **324**: 332–5

12.2 (a) T   (b) T   (c) F   (d) T   (e) T

Fatovich DM (2002) Recent developments: Emergency medicine. *Br Med J* **324**: 958–62

12.3 (a) F   (b) F   (c) T   (d) T   (e) T

Fatovich DM (2002) Recent developments: Emergency medicine. *Br Med J* **324**: 958–62

Cummings P, McKnight B, Rivara FP *et al* (2002)Association of driver air bags with driver
    fatality: a matched cohort study. *Br Med J* **324**: 1119–22

Halman SI, Chipman M, Parkin PC *et al* (2002) Are seat belt restraints as effective in school
    age children as in adults? A prospective crash study. *Br Med J* **324**: 1123–5

Connor J, Norton R, Ameratunga S *et al* (2002) Driver sleepiness and risk of serious injury to
    car occupants: population based case controlled study. *Br Med J* **324**: 1125–8

Hippisley-Cox J, Groom L, Kendrick D *et al* (2002) Cross sectional survey of socioeconomic
    variations in severity and mechanism of childhood injuries in Trent 1992–7. *Br Med J*
    324: 1132–4

Coats TJ, Davies G (2002) Prehospital care for road traffic casualties. *Br Med J* **324**: 1135–8

12.4 (a) T   (b) F   (c) T   (d) F   (e) F

Gibbons RV, Vaughn DW (2002) Clinical review: Dengue: an escalating problem. *Br Med J*
    324: 1563–6

12.5 (a) T   (b) T   (c) F   (d) F   (e) T

Zuckerman JN (2002) Recent developments: Travel medicine. *Br Med J* **325**: 260–4

12.6 (a) T (b) T (c) F (d) T (e) F

Beckingham IJ, Bornman PC (2001) ABC of liver, pancreas, and biliary system: Acute pancreatitis. *Br Med J* **322**: 595–8

12.7 (a) T (b) T (c) T (d) F (e) T

Fatovich DM (2002) Recent developments: Emergency medicine. *Br Med J* **324**: 958–62

Australasian College for Emergency Medicine, Royal Australian and New Zealand College of Psychiatrists (2000) Guidelines for the management of deliberate self harm in young people. In: Melbourne, Victoria: Australasian College for Emergency Medicine, Royal Australian and New Zealand College of Psychiatrists www.acem.org.au/open/documents/youthsuicide.pdf

12.8 (a) F (b) F (c) F (d) T (e) T

American College of Surgeons, Committee on Trauma (1997) *Advanced Trauma Life Support, Student Manual*. 6th edition. American College of Surgeons, Chicago

12.9 (a) F (b) F (c) T (d) F (e) T

Maas R, Ventura R, Kretzschmar C *et al* (2003) Syncope, driving recommendations, and clinical reality: survey of patients. *Br Med J* **326**: 21

12.10 (a) T (b) F (c) T (d) T (e) F

British Medical Association (2003) *British National Formulary*. 46 edn. British Medical Association and Royal Pharmaceutical Society of Great Britain, London

12.11 (a) T (b) F (c) F (d) T (e) T

Reece J, Price J, eds (2000) *ABC of Asthma*. Fourth edition. BMJ Books, London

12.12 (a) F (b) F (c) F (d) T (e) T

British Medical Association (2003) *British National Formulary*. 46 edn. British Medical Association and Royal Pharmaceutical Society of Great Britain, London

12.13 (a) F (b) F (c) T (d) T (e) T

Lawrence N, Watts J, Harrington R *et al* (1997) *Handbook of Emergencies in General Practice*. Second edition. Oxford University Press, Oxford

12.14 (a) T (b) F (c) T (d) T (e) T

Ewan P (1998) ABC of allergies. *Br Med J* **316**: 1442–5

12.15   (a) T   (b) T   (c) F   (d) F   (e) T
Fennerty T (1997) Fortnightly review: The diagnosis of pulmonary embolism. *Br Med J* **314**:
425

12.16   (a) T   (b) F   (c) T   (d) T   (e) F
Jeffrey SLA, Cubison TCS, Greenaway C *et al* (2000) Lesson of the week: Warming milk-a
preventable cause of scalds in children. *Br Med J* **320**: 235

12.17   (a) T   (b) F   (c) F   (d) F   (e) T
Brenner R (2002) Childhood drowning is a global concern. *Br Med J* **324**: 1049–50

EMQ 1

1	increase
2	lowest
3	anxiety
4	reassurance
5	increase
6	heart
7	overestimation
8	underestimation
9	overestimation
10	underestimation
11	undercuffing
12	overcuffing
13	white coat
14	ambulatory blood pressure measurement.

Beevers G, Lip GYH, O'Brien E (2001) ABC of hypertension. Blood pressure measurement:
Sphygmomanometry: factors common to all techniques. *Br Med J* **322**: 981–5

EMQ 2

1	D
2	A
3	B
4	E
5	C

UK Prospective Diabetes Study Group (1998) Tight blood pressure control and risk of
macrovascular and microvascular complications in type 2 diabetes. UKPDS 38. *Br Med J*
317: 703–13
National Institute of Clinical Excellence (NICE) guidelines: Type 2 diabetes-management of
blood pressure and lipids. London, October 2002. www.nice.org.uk

Ramsey LE, Williams B, Johnston DG *et al* (1999) Guidelines for the management of hypertension: Report of the third working party of the British Hypertension Society. *J Hypetens* **13**: 569–92

EMQ 3

1	K
2	H
3	I
4	D
5	L
6	B
7	F
8	E

Khaw PT, Elkington AR (1999) *ABC of Eyes*. Third edition. BMJ books, London

EMQ 4

1	G
2	E
3	B
4	H
5	C
6	D
7	A
8	I
9	F

McLatchie GR, Lennox CME, Eds (1993) *The Soft Tissues: Trauma and Sports Injuries*. Butterworth Heinemann, Oxford

Aliotta P, Baustian G, Birnbaumer D *et al*, eds (2003) *PDxMD Rheumatology*. Steven Merahn, Philadelphia

EMQ 5

1	D
2	C
3	G
4	F
5	E
6	A
7	B

Linde K, Ramirez G, Mulrow CD *et al* (1996) St John's wort for depression—An overview and meta-analysis of randomised clinical trials. *Br Med J* **313**: 253–8

Melchart D, Linde K, Fischer P *et al* (1999) *Echinacea for preventing and treating the common cold*. In: Cochrane Collaboration. The Cochrane Library. Issue 3. Update Software, Oxford

Wilt TJ, Ishani A, Stark G *et al* (1998) Saw palmetto extracts for treatment of benign prostatic hyperplasia: A systematic review. *JAMA* **280**: 1604–1609

Vickers A, Zollman C (1999) Clinical review: Herbal medicine. *Br Med J* **319**: 1050–3

EMQ 6

1   C, D, H
2   A, F, I
3   B, E, G

Jones J, Boorman J, Cann P *et al* (2001) British Society of Gastroenterology guidelines for the management of the irritable bowel syndrome. *Gut* **49**(3): 455

Forbes A, Gabe S, Lennard-Jones J *et al* (2003) Screening and surveillance for asymptomatic colorectal cancer in IBD. *Gut* **52**(5): 769–9

Hardy R, Meltzer S, Jankowski J (2000) ABC of colorectal cancer: Molecular basis for risk factors. *Br Med J* **321**: 886–9

Jones R (2002) Commentary: Functional abdominal pain: another unexplained physical symptom. *Int J Epidemiol* **31**: 1225–6

Guthrie E, Thompson D (2002) ABC of psychological medicine: Abdominal pain and functional gastrointestinal disorders. *Br Med J* **325**: 701–3

EMQ 7

1   arterial thromboembolism
2   chronic liver disease
3   obesity
4   deep vein thrombosis
5   androgenic
6   deep vein thrombosis
7   oestrogenic
8   breast
9   cervix
10   ovary
11   endometrium
12   triphasic
13   tricycle
14   premenstrual tension
15   nausea
16   vaginal discharge without infection
17   hirsutism
18   loss of libido

Guillebaud J (1999) *Contraception: Your questions answered*. Third edition. Churchill Livingstone, London

EMQ 8

1	E
2	A
3	A, B, C
4	B, F, G
5	E
6	C
7	C, G
8	B, D, F

Klippel JH, Dippe PA (1997) *Rheumatology*. Second edition. Mosby, London
ISBN 0 7234 2405 5

EMQ 9

1	A, B
2	B
3	E, F
4	A,C,G
5	B, H
6	D, F, H

Klippel JH, Dippe PA (1997) *Rheumatology*. Second edition. Mosby, London
ISBN 0 7234 2405 5

EMQ 10

1	A
2	A
3	A, C
4	B
5	A
6	B, D, E
7	C
8	E, F

Rowlands S, Devalia H, Smith C *et al* (2001) Otitis externa in UK general practice: A survey using the UK General Practice Research Database. *Br Med J* **51**:533–7

Browning G (2002) In: Barton S, ed, *Clinical Evidence*. BMJ Publishing Group, London 1159–60

T Aung, Mulley G (2002) Ten-minute consultation: Removal of ear wax. *Br Med J* **325**: 27

EMQ 11

1	A
2	A, C, H
3	B, D
4	A, C, F, H
5	B, F, H
6	E, F, G
7	D, I, J

MacFarlane J, Prewett J, Rose D *et al* (1997) Prospective case-control study of role of infection in patients who reconsult after initial antibiotic treatment for lower respiratory tract infection in primary care. *Br Med J* **315**: 1206–10

EMQ 12

1	A, B, F
2	A, E, I, L
3	A, D, F
4	F
5	A, B, F
6	I, L
7	I
8	B, I

Weller R, O'Callaghan C, MacSween R *et al* (1999) Scarring in molluscum contagiosum: comparison of physical expression and phenol ablation. *Br Med J* **319**: 1540

Crawford F, Hart R, Bell-Syer S *et al* (2001) Extracts from Clinical Evidence: Athlete's foot and fungally infected toenails. *Br Med J* **322**: 288–9

Webster G, Poyner T, Cunliffe B (2002) Acne vulgaris. Commentary: A UK primary care perspective on treating acne. *Br Med J* **325**: 475–9

Gibbs S, Harvey I, Sterling J *et al* (2002) Local treatments for cutaneous warts: Systematic review. Commentary: Systematic reviewers face challenges from varied study designs. *Br Med J* **325**: 461

Bayat A, McGrouther DA, Ferguson MWJ (2003) Skin scarring. *Br Med J* **326**: 88–92

Friedmann P (1998) ABC of allergies: Allergy and the skin 2. Contact and atopic eczema. *Br Med J* **316**: 1226

Biographies

Mei Ling Denney has been a full-time GP principal in Peterborough for many years, and now has a 'portfolio' GP career working in general practice and medical education. She is interested in various aspects of primary care education, assessment and appraisal. At present, she is a VTS Course Organiser, examiner for summative assessment and the MRCGP exam panel. She teaches on a number of courses, including exam preparation and work at the Universities of Cambridge and Oxford.

Christopher Hand has been a GP in Bungay, Suffolk, for twenty-seven years and is a fellow of the Royal College of Physicians and the Royal College of General Practitioners. He has been involved in GP education since 1980. He has been a GP trainer, a course organiser and an associate adviser. In 1992, he completed an MSc in general practice at Guy's and St Thomas' Hospitals. In 1994, he joined the University of East Anglia and helped to set up the MSc in Health Sciences. More recently, he was a member of the team that successfully bid for UEA to become one of the four new UK. medical schools, and now is actively involved with the UEA undergraduate curriculum[1]. His research interests include patients' beliefs about inhaler treatment for asthma, and SHO training.

Amanda Howe graduated from Cambridge and the Royal London in 1979, and spent twenty years in Sheffield before joining the University of East Anglia as its first Professor of Primary Care. She is still a practising GP, but became increasingly involved in university medical education and latterly research, now holding both a Masters in Education and an MD. Her research interests include professional development of students, innovative assessment, and the role of the public in improving health care. She is also a Fellow of the Royal College of General Practitioners, and was Chair of their Research Group from 2000–2003.

Judith Neaves is a practising GP, working variously in Surrey, the Outer Hebrides, and now rural Norfolk. Her involvement in education stems from 1994 when she became a GP trainer. She is an examiner for the Royal College of General Practitioners, and involved in undergraduate teaching at the medical school at UEA. She is a Musculoskeletal Physician and Osteopath, having an MSc in this field from University College, London.

---

1. UEA undergraduate curriculum, modelled on 200 clinical presentations.